Get Set for Nursing

T0173403

Titles in the GET SET FOR UNIVERSITY series:

Get Set for American Studies
ISBN 0 7486 1692 6

Get Set for Study in the UK
ISBN 0 7486 1810 4

Get Set for English Language
ISBN 0 7486 1544 X

Get Set for Nursing
ISBN 0 7486 1956 9

Get Set for English Literature
ISBN 0 7486 1537 7

*Get Set for Communication
 Studies*
ISBN 0 7486 2029 X

Get Set for Philosophy
ISBN 0 7486 1657 8

Get Set for Sociology
ISBN 0 7486 2019 2

Get Set for Politics
ISBN 0 7486 1545 8

Get Set for Nursing

Graeme D. Smith

Edinburgh University Press

© Graeme D. Smith, 2004

Edinburgh University Press Ltd
22 George Square, Edinburgh

Typeset in Sabon
by Hewer Text Ltd, Edinburgh, and
printed and bound in Finland by
WS Bookwell

A CIP record for this book is
available from the British Library

ISBN 0 7486 1956 9 (paperback)

The right of Graeme D. Smith
to be identified as author of this work
has been asserted in accordance with
the Copyright, Designs and Patents Act 1988.

CONTENTS

PART I: A GUIDE TO NURSING

PART II: STUDY SKILLS

FOREWORD

Choosing a career in nursing can be one of the most challenging and rewarding experiences life can offer. However, nursing is a broad church with many fields of practice and many disciplines to draw upon in order to understand the unique nature of the human response to illness. The twenty-first century sees a time when nursing is changing quite dramatically particularly in the area of autonomous professional practice. More and more patients receive their care within a nurse-led context which formerly might have been the preserve of the medical profession. Equally, care that in the past was always within the hospital context is now increasingly in the community. What is universally recognised is that nursing is a complex profession that has at its heart the needs of patients and clients whilst always working alongside other health-care professionals – the multidisciplinary team. Nursing is a profession that needs, from the moment of entry, a commitment to ongoing learning. The nursing knowledge and skills that we value so highly are always being developed as new evidence from research takes us forward.

This short text looks to share with those who might be thinking about a career as a nurse the opportunity to gain an insight into the fundamental elements of nursing practice. The reader will see that nursing is not merely about procedures, anatomy or disorders, it is about being with patients and understanding them as whole people within a family and social context and how this impacts on them in relation to health and illness experiences. In other words, holistic care.

There is no denying that as a society we need more nurses, but we need nurses who understand the career they have chosen and *Get Set for Nursing* will help prospective nursing students appreciate, beyond the stereotypical images, the real nature of nursing such that they might make an informed decision – something we always look to ensure in our patients.

Tonks Fawcett
Head of Nursing Studies
University of Edinburgh

ACKNOWLEDGEMENTS

I would like to acknowledge the many people who were important in the process of completing this text. First, I would like to recognise several students and staff who have made helpful contributions to this book: Sarah Baggaley, Pearl Culbert, Yvonne Freer, Alison Jarvis, Anne Rowatt, Deborah Tomlinson and Roger Watson. Particular thanks to Tonks Fawcett for her encouragement and helpful feedback along the way. Thanks to Gillian Kidd for her help with medical illustration. Once again many thanks to Linda for her secretarial skills. Special thanks to my parents for helping me to find a correct place for everything.

PREFACE

The knowledge base of students entering university courses to study nursing can differ widely. Some students may have just completed their secondary education, others may have recently completed a further education course, whilst others may not have studied for a long time. Additionally, some nursing students may have had limited exposure to the core subjects they will encounter: nursing, biology and social sciences.

With this in mind, it is the aim of this text to provide students with a basic introduction and overview of the core subjects they will encounter in the common foundation of pre-registration nursing programmes. Despite the fact that nursing courses vary between institutions throughout the UK, all courses must satisfy the requirements of the common foundation programme. The first year of all pre-registration nursing courses is a common foundation programme, which introduces the student to the basic principles of nursing. At the end of the common foundation programme the student nurse will choose to specialise in either adult nursing, children's nursing, mental-health nursing or in learning-disability nursing.

This book is relatively brief and only 'scratches the surface' of some of the material that may be encountered in the common foundation programme. As such, this is not intended to be a comprehensive overview and nursing students will be provided with set texts to read as they enter the common foundation programme. It is hoped that this text will complement these. Additional reading lists are provided throughout this text.

Each of the chapters in both Parts I and II discusses a particular topic of relevance to nursing studies. In Chapter 1, nursing is examined; from the philosophy of nursing, to the five stages of the nursing process, nursing models, to the inter-professional role of nurses. Chapter 2 relates to the importance of biological sciences within nursing. This theme is continued in Chapter 3, which examines the relevance of social sciences, psychology and sociology. Some of the main theoretical issues in nurse education having been introduced in the first three chapters, Chapter 4 attempts to link this theory to practice by covering some of the clinical skills required in nursing care. Student nurses will be required to record blood pressure accurately or to understand the relevance of measuring glucose levels in urine. Chapter 5 highlights safety issues in nursing. Finally, Part II covers study skills. As university students it is important to be aware of the study skills that are required to aid preparation for exams, write essays and get the most from your lectures.

INTRODUCTION

WHY GO TO UNIVERSITY?

You may be a seeker after knowledge and/or you may be going for the social life and/or you may be going because it is expected of you. Whatever your reasons, graduation day comes and you have to find a job. You would expect a university degree to improve your job prospects, but have you ever wondered why? Even with a general Arts degree, the market for professional philosophers and literary critics is very limited. What employers are actually looking for are transferable skills and you have to make sure your prospective employer knows that you have them.

General Transferable Skills

- University graduates are self-motivating.

- They are good at time-management.

- They can work under pressure.

- They can meet deadlines.

- They have learned from their tutorials how to be team-players and how to work as part of a group.

- They have shown that they are well-rounded individuals by taking an active part in at least one of the sporting, social or intellectual activities offered by university societies or clubs.

WHY CHOSE NURSING?

The best reason for choosing nursing is because you like it, but it brings its own transferable skills bonuses which often go unrecognised and which will be of lifelong service to you. Job prospects are excellent in both the public and private sectors, regardless of whether you choose to train as an adult, a mental-health, learning-difficulites or children's nurse.

Transferable Skills

Studying at university will also:

- Enhance your written communication skills. You will know how to write clearly, concisely and, above all, accurately and unambiguously. You will also be adept at matching the level of formality to suit different types of readers.

- Enhance your reading skills. You will be able to analyse non-literary texts and make sense of the most difficult constructions. You will even be able to spot when and why a very wise-sounding text may make no sense at all. You will read between the lines.

- Enhance your oral and aural skills. You will have confidence in your own accent. You will not prejudge people because their accents are different from yours. You will understand how accommodation and turn-taking work in conversations and people will find you easy to talk to.

- Enhance your thinking skills. Few subjects bring together the many different ways of thinking that nursing demands. You need to think clearly, methodically and logically. You will be able to seek out and evaluate evidence.

A SPECIAL WORD TO MATURE STUDENTS

Some mature students worry too much. If you are a mature student coming to university for the first time, you may have many problems to contend with that students straight from school do not have. You may have family commitments, perhaps even young children and all the worries about child care that parenthood entails. Your university may provide good-quality, low-cost child care. This is worth finding out about. You may have got out of the habit of studying, writing essays and sitting exams and the young students seem incredibly self-confident and knowledgeable. You will soon get back into the way of studying and you would not have been admitted to university if you did not have the ability to succeed; so there is no reason to compare your talents unfavourably with those of younger students. For some reason, many mature students feel that they have to do better than the younger students to prove to themselves that they can do as well. If this sounds like you, calm down. Your maturity gives you extra skills, particularly in time management and communication. It is always a joy to teach mature students because of their high level of motivation and because they ask lots of questions. If any domestic crises should occur, or if you are having difficulty with any aspect of study, you will find that members of staff are very understanding and supportive.

PART I
A Guide to Nursing

1 WHAT IS NURSING?

Everyone enters nursing with a wide range of personal beliefs
and values. These develop from our own life experiences and
are influenced by our moral upbringing, ethnic origin, educational opportunity and religious beliefs. In addition to these
life experiences, as a student nurse you will be exposed to a
range of professional beliefs and values, which will be accom-
modated into the way you practise as a nurse. From reading
textbooks, from lecturers and from clinically based nurses,
you will encounter different ways of looking at nursing.

Professional nursing beliefs and values are defined by the
Nursing and Midwifery Council (NMC). The NMC has
recently replaced the United Kingdom Central Council for
Nursing, Midwifery and Health Visiting (UKCC) as the stat-
utory body responsible for regulating nursing education and
entry. These professional codes of conduct clearly identify the
standards of practice expected from nurses and provide nurses
with a baseline of values and beliefs which are deemed
appropriate at different times. Indeed, the NMC has the power
to sanction any nurses who contravene its codes, even in their
private lives. Therefore anyone calling themselve a nurse,
midwife or health visitor is assumed to behave in the way
of a registered practitioner, as set out in the Code of Professional Conduct.

Groups of nurses working together within a clinical area
will deliver care with a shared philosophy. The use of the word
'philosophy' in nursing tends to refer to a way of doing things,
underpinned by a written statement of beliefs and values. All
clinical areas providing placements for student nurses are
required to have a nursing philosophy. This philosophy
should include an explanation of how and why things are
done, a statement of intent and belief, a statement of the

purpose of the organisation and individuals, and a consideration of the role of nursing. To be effective, a nursing philosophy must have practical applications to the area for which it
was written and must reflect the current practices that occur.
For student nurses, the philosophy of a clinical area helps to
introduce the basis for the development of nursing care in that
clinical setting. Models of nursing are examined later in this
chapter.

TYPES OF NURSES
All nurses focus on the needs of the individual, rather than
specific illnesses or conditions. Nursing in the twenty-first
century involves:

- ensuring the promotion and delivery of top-quality, evidence-based care

- ensuring the empowerment of patients, with promotion of
  the ability to care for themselves

- ensuring patient access to appropriate health-care services

- co-ordination of nursing care throughout the patient journey

- effective teamwork across a variety of professional groups
  and agencies

- the ongoing development and improvement of nursing and
  midwifery practice.

The variety of roles in nursing profession is vast. As a nurse
there are opportunities to work in hospitals, the community,
health centres, nursing homes, occupational health services,
voluntary-organisation-run hospices, residential care and the
pharmaceutical industry. Nurses also work in university education, in the prison service and for the armed forces.

Nurses qualify from one of four branches of nurse education: adult, children, mental health and learning disability.

Adult nursing

Nurses trained on the adult branch of nursing are by far the largest group of nurses. Adult nurses can work in hospitals or in the community and care for, support and educate people of all ages. Adult nurses often take additional courses once they have qualified to specialise. These courses include cancer care, accident and emergency, critical care, district nursing and health visiting.

Children's nursing

Nurses who qualify on the children's branch of nursing work with 0 to 18-year-olds in a variety of settings from specialist baby care units in children's hospitals to adolescent services. Children react to illness and disease in a very different manner to adults, which is why they need to be cared for by specially trained nurses, who understand their particular needs. Children's nurses also support, educate and advise parents of children and other close relatives. Once qualified as a children's nurse it is possible to specialise in a variety of clinical areas in hospitals and in the community, such as burns and plastics, critical care, cancer care and child protection.

Mental-health nursing

The vast majority of people with mental-health problems are based in the community. Therefore mental-health nurses work closely with general practitioners (GPs), psychiatrists and social workers to co-ordinate the care of individuals with mental-health problems. Nurses plan and deliver nursing care for people in their own homes or in specialist hospital services.

Within mental-health nursing it is possible to specialise in areas such as rehabilitation, child and adolescent mental health and substance misuse. Mental-health nurses may undertake specific training in therapies such as psychotherapy and cognitive behavioural therapy.

Learning-disabilities nursing

Nurses who qualify in this field of nursing help people with learning disabilities to live independent and fulfilling lives. About 2–3 per cent of the UK population has a learning disability. Caring for those with learning disabilities usually involves the nurse working in supported accommodation; typically three to four individuals with learning disability live together in a flat or house, with 24-hour support. Some nurses work with individuals who require intensive support in specialist secure units for learning disabilities. Learning-disability nurses specialise in areas such as epilepsy management or working with sensory impairment.

Nurses and midwives play a dynamic and vital role in improving health and delivering health services. Several short accounts illustrate the diversity of roles in nursing.

DISTRICT NURSE

'A District Nurse is a registered nurse with a qualification in community health studies/district nursing. District Nurses assess, provide and manage skilled nursing care to people in their own homes. They undertake complex assessments of the health and nursing needs of patients whose nursing needs can best be met at home and work with them and their carers to promote self-care and a return to independence where possible. The District Nurse leads a team of registered nurses and nursing auxiliaries and is usually attached to a GP practice. District Nurses collaborate with a wide range of specialist health staff both in the community and in the hospital. They work at the boundary of health and social care delivery, so they make a major contribution to the multidisciplinary assessment of patients, formulation of care packages and liaison with other service providers. District Nurses are experts in wound assessment and care. They have skills in acute and chronic disease management as well as palliative and terminal care. District Nurses are involved in the prescribing of drugs and health-care products as well as the administration of treatments such as enteral feeding, phlebotomy, doppler assessment, ear syringing and ECG. The majority of a District Nurse's caseload are patients aged sixty-five years and over. A fundamental part of district nursing is promoting healthy lifestyles and health education and teaching as well as supporting the informal carer of the patient. District Nurses are often an essential ingredient in the complex arrangement of support needed to sustain people in their own homes.'

NURSE PRACTITIONER

'I think I am very lucky. I am a nurse practitioner (GI [gastro intestinal]) and I love my job.

Having reached my middle years, with some grace, I hope, and some disgrace, thank goodness, every working day brings new challenges and experiences.

My job has evolved and developed over the last four years. For example, I have recently completed nurse endoscopist training in flexible sigmoidoscopy. This was probably the hardest thing I have taken on, but I accepted the challenge and have succeeded.

The hands-on patient contact is something I value greatly, as well as the teaching component of my work.

Extended roles mean more autonomy for practitioners. This is a mixed blessing. One's decision-making skills are certainly honed, and the knowledge base on which the decisions are made must be continually updated.

There are times when I could see it all far enough, telling myself that I want a job where people are not placing such demands on me. Some days it feels like everyone wants a piece [of me]. A registrar would surely have carried out the work I do now, a decade ago. We nurse practitioners are certainly a valuable resource.

Other times, when going about my working day, I marvel at how far nurses have come since I first proudly put on my starched hat and apron all those years ago.'

HEALTH VISITOR

'Health visitors, increasingly known as public health practitioners, are registered nurses with a community health studies/ public health nursing qualification. The principles of health visiting are:

1. The search for health needs
2. Stimulation of an awareness of health needs
3. Influences on policies affecting health
4. The facilitation of health-enhancing activities. (CETHV 1977; Twinn and Cowley 1992)

Health visitors usually are based in a GP practice, with a major focus of their work being a universal service to families with preschool children. Through assessment, support and advice, working in partnership with families, they promote child health and development, improve maternal health and well-being and enhance parenting skills and the home environment. Health visitors visit families antenatally and after delivery take over from the community midwife. Work is undertaken in both the home and clinic setting with a core programme of childhood immunisations and developmental surveillance. Child protection, within a multidisciplinary and legal framework, is a fundamental aspect of their work.

Recent government policy aimed at tackling poverty, social exclusion and inequalities in access to health care sees health visitors as key to advancing this agenda through their expert knowledge of communities and their health needs, combined with their skill at communicating with a variety of professionals and voluntary organisations across the public and private sectors. Health visitors participate in an increasing range of community programmes including antenatal education, parenting classes, sleep clinics, postnatal depression groups, healthy eating, smoking cessation, baby massage and Sure Start programmes.

Health visitors are uniquely placed to contribute to the health of individuals, families and communities in the twenty-first century.'

MIDWIFE

What it is to be a midwife

'A midwife gives information and offers support and care to women and their families before and throughout pregnancy as well as during the birth of the baby and up to twenty-eight days afterwards. The "care" setting may be the woman's home, the General Practitioner's surgery or the hospital. Most midwives work within a team of other health professionals but there are those who choose to work independently from the National Health Service.

The work of a midwife involves more than being only with well women, their babies and families. You will be called upon to care for women with pregnancy-related problems as well as those unrelated to but compounded by the pregnancy; skills in nursing the woman who has had major surgery are also required. Equally, not all babies are well and you will have responsibility for detecting problems and managing these babies.

Being a midwife requires many special qualities. In-depth knowledge and understanding, empathy and communication skills are all essential. Appreciation that the delivery of health care is more than just the giving of physical attention is required. This is especially important when considering the many social and cultural differences that exist within today's society and that influence health and health needs.'

How to become a midwife

'There are two educational programmes that you can undertake to become a midwife. There is the three-year programme, sometimes referred to as direct entry, or the eighteen-month programme for those who already have a nursing qualification. Both programmes offer a mix of theory and practice and, depending on the institution, may be offered at degree or diploma level.'

CHILDREN'S NURSE

'Questions all children's nurses have to face at some point: "How do you handle it, working with children who are sick? I would get too attached. Isn't it sad?"

No, it isn't sad!

I remember as a student children's nurse we all wore badges that said "Sick Children: It takes a special kind of nurse". We were proud of these badges while at the same time slightly embarrassed, realising that we weren't special at all. The children are special; the families are special. Children and their families cope with accidents, illness and disease in various ways but they always manage to come through the ordeal.

Nursing sick children is based on a philosophy of family-centred care. The family can include parents, siblings, grandparents and even any other significant people in the child's life. The family is encouraged to be involved in caring for their child.

Children have their own needs for nursing care. Primarily it is important to know and understand the normal growth and development of children. Then we have some guidance when something goes wrong. Many illnesses and diseases are exclusive to children. Children can deteriorate much more rapidly than adults, so nurses must be aware of this and take it into consideration when planning care. We cannot learn one expected normal heart rate, respiratory rate or blood pressure for children; values vary usually depending on the child's age. Children can also get better more quickly than adults – once they are feeling physically better they can get up and around, often forgetting a very serious illness or accident.

We may cry occasionally on the way home about a sad scene that we were involved in, but often we have been witness to amazing bravery; discharged children who have made a complete recovery; or just made a parent understand a bit more about what is happening. Nursing children is sometimes exhausting, sometimes frustrating, but usually rewarding.'

ACADEMIC NURSE

'An increasing number of nurses work in universities where they contribute to the teaching of nurses and carry out research into nursing. After training as a nurse and working with older people in the NHS, I left my job as a charge nurse in a busy unit for older people and became a lecturer in nursing. I had previous experience as a biologist and already had a Ph.D. in biochemistry. I readily moved into teaching biology to undergraduate pre-registration nurses and established a programme of research into the feeding problems of older people with dementia. This work was a continuation of my clinical work and the academic environment gave me the time and resources to follow my interests and to give something back to the NHS.

Currently I work as a professor of nursing, a role in which I provide academic leadership to colleagues in my university and in my local NHS Trusts. Part of my salary is paid by the NHS and this ensures that I have regular contact with nurses in practice from whom I learn about the issues they face. Being an academic has not divorced me from practice and, while I have no direct responsibility for patient care, through my teaching and research I continue to make a contribution to patient care and the development of the next generation of practitioners.'

REFLECTION ON THE NURSE'S ROLE

'I decided at the age of fourteen that I wanted to be a nurse. At the age of eighteen I was very fortunate to begin my nursing studies and training at the University of Edinburgh. After four, hard-working but also fantastic years I finally became a registered nurse!

I have now been a qualified nurse for nine years, working in the area of surgery. I can honestly say that I love my job and can't think of any other career I would rather have. Like most jobs you can have good and bad days and nursing is no different in this respect. When you know that you have played a part in assisting a patient on the road to recovery, there is no better feeling.

There are so many different areas and specialities that a nurse can choose to work in. As a nurse you have the option to work in as many or as few areas as you want. I also think that if you specialise in one particular area you continually learn new aspects of that speciality every day. That is one of the many reasons that I enjoy my job so much.

At the end of the day your job is what you make of it and nursing is exactly the same. It is such a rewarding career and you get the opportunity to work with so many people (for example physiotherapists and occupational therapists) and you get the chance to care for a wide variety of patients.

To summarise, being a nurse is rewarding, exhausting, sociable, a continual learning experience, brilliant!'

BECOMING A STUDENT NURSE

Personal qualities

Nursing attracts people with all kinds of personalities from all sorts of backgrounds. You will need to be non-judgemental and a good communicator with the ability to listen, empathise and provide support. If you enjoy working with people and would like to make a difference to their lives, the nursing profession has a lot to offer you. To enter the nursing profession you must by law be aged seventeen years and six months (17 years in Scotland) at the start of the course. Acceptance on any university-based nursing course will depend on several factors, including your health, past convictions and academic qualifications.

You will be required to complete a health questionnaire when you apply for nursing or midwifery training. Acceptance on a nursing course usually involves a satisfactory health clearance. Students must also declare any previous criminal convictions or police record.

Qualifications

The following are the minimum entry requirements for nursing courses:

- 5 GCSE/GCE O levels, grade C or above (including English); or

- 5 CSEs Grade 1; or

- 5 SCEs Grade 1; or

- 5 SCE ordinary, grades A–C (Scotland); or

- GNVQ Advanced level or NVQ level 3; or

- an Access to Higher Education Course.

However, universities usually require students to hold much more than the minimum. These requirements vary between institutions. Further information on the application process for nursing is available from the following organisations:

NHS Careers
PO BOX 376
Bristol BS99 322
Tel: 0845 60 60 655
E-mail:
    advice@nhscareers.nhs.uk
Website:
    www.nhscareers.nhs.uk

NHS Education for Scotland
66 Rose Street
Edinburgh EH2 2NN
Tel: 0131 220 8666
E-mail:
    careers@nes.scot.nhs.uk
Website:
    www.nbs.org.uk

NHS Professions Wales
Golate House
101 St Mary Street
Cardiff CF1 1DX
Tel: 02920 261400
Website: www.wnb.org.uk

NIPEC Queen's University
    Belfast
University Road
Belfast BT7 1NN
Tel: 028 9024 5133
Website: www.qub.ac.uk

Funding

Funding is always an issue for prospective nursing students. Students who undertake a NHS-funded degree course will receive a non-means-tested bursary. At the time of writing, this currently stands at £5,432 per annum (£6,382 in London). As each individual's personal and financial circumstances vary, it is suggested that detailed information on funding is obtained from one of the following organisations:

The NHS Student Grants
    Unit
Room 212 Government
    Buildings
Norcross
Blackpool FY5 3TA
Tel: 01253 333314

The Students Awards
    Agency for Scotland
3 Redheughs Rigg
South Gyle
Edinburgh EH12 9HH
Tel: 0131 476 8212

The NHS (Wales) Student Awards
Human Resources Division
National Assembly for Wales
Cathays Park
Cardiff CF10 3NQ
Tel: 02920 82 6886

Department of Higher and Further Education
Student Support Branch
4th Floor Adelaide House
39–49 Adelaide Street
Belfast BT2 8FD
Tel: 028 9025 7777

Application

There is a central application for both degree and diploma nursing courses. To apply for a degree programme you need to apply to:

The University and College Admissions Service (UCAS)
Barn Lane
Cheltenham
Gloucestershire GL52 3LZ
Tel: 01242 227788 (for application packs)
     01242 222444 (general enquiries)

For diploma programmes you need to apply to:

The Nursing and Midwifery Admission Service (NMAS)
Rosehill, New Barn Lane
Cheltenham
Gloucestershire GL52 3LZ
Tel: 01242 223707 (for application pack)
     01242 544949 (general enquiries)

THE NURSING PROCESS

To ensure that nursing care is planned and delivered effectively a structured approach called the 'nursing process' is used. This is a planned problem-solving approach to meet an individual's health-care and nursing requirements. It enables nurses to plan care on an individual basis and provides a scientific approach towards nursing. The student nurse should be aware that the nursing process is not undertaken only once, as the needs of the patient will constantly change and the nurse must respond appropriately. For example, if an individual is in pain, it is not enough to make an assessment of the situation and plan an intervention; the nurse needs to make a reassessment following evaluation of the pain-relieving intervention. The nursing process is therefore a dynamic and ongoing cyclic process; it is not a one-off activity.

The importance of understanding and implementing a systematic approach to the provision of nursing care is of vital importance to student nurses. Nurses are accountable for the care that they deliver and the nursing process provides them with a problem-solving framework to document their actions in a logical and rational manner. Failure to keep an accurate record of care can lead to a breakdown in the quality of nursing care provided.

There is some debate within the nursing profession as to how many stages exist within the nursing process. Some suggest four and others five. For the purpose of this text, a five-stage process will be adopted to enable the student nurse to identify the patient's nursing diagnosis in order to plan the most appropriate care.

The whole sequence of the nursing process, therefore, is:

- assessment: collection of objective and subjective data

- nursing diagnosis: identification of potential or actual health problems

- planning nursing care: plan the care or intervention to resolve the problem

- implementation: delivery of nursing interventions

- evaluation: appraisal of the effectiveness of the intervention.

As mentioned earlier, the nursing process should not be viewed as a linear process.

Stage 1: Assessment

Assessment is not an easy process and it usually involves collecting information from a variety of sources. These sources include: the patient, relatives of the patient, previous nursing records and medical notes. The structure of the assessment interview should cover the following areas:

- demographic details

- reason for admission

- past medical history

- family history

- the ability to meet the activities of daily living (see below)

- psychological or social factors that may affect health (psychosocial factors)

- physical assessment of vital signs (e.g. temperature, pulse and blood pressure).

When admitting a patient into your nursing care there are certain specific assessment activities that need to be undertaken. As these are completed the required information will be obtained. The initial of these activities relates to first impressions that you notice about the patient. When you first set eyes on the patient you will already be observing and assessing that individual. Does the patient look in pain or discomfort? Are they anxious or distressed? Has he or she any obvious physical injuries or abnormalities? These initial informal observations can give the nurse some subtle clues about a patient's current health status prior to the assessment interview.

This formal assessment interview will involve a range of skills:

- listening

- observing

- use of non-verbal communication

- open and closed questions

- physical examination

- objective measurements.

It is very important to introduce yourself to patients when you first meet and to address them by their preferred title; the nurse should give the patient the opportunity to choose what he or she would like to be called. If patients are unfamiliar with the health-care environment, the nurse should try to reduce anxiety by explaining who will be caring for them from the multidisciplinary team and how to distinguish between the uniforms of the variety of staff that may be encountered. At this early stage the nurse should determine if there are any potential communication barriers. For example, the patient may not speak English or may have a speech or hearing difficulty. Prior to the assessment interview the nurse should prepare by gathering key biographical details from the medical notes, such information as date of birth, address and contact number of the next of kin; these should be verified with the

patient. If possible the assessment interview should be conducted in a comfortable and quiet place. The nurse should aim
to provide a calm, unhurried and non-judgemental atmosphere for the assessment. A non-judgemental atmosphere
involves not showing disgust, shock or anger with any of
the information that patients provide about their lifestyle (e.g.
heavy drinking or sexual orientation). Patients are far more
likely to relax and provide all the information that is required
if time and attention is given to them.

Be aware that some nursing/medical jargon may limit the
patient's understanding of the questions you are asking, so it is
better to use lay language and terms. For example, 'Have you
had a trace of your heart activity recently?' Is clearer for the
patient than 'Have you had an ECG recently?'.

One of the most important features of assessment relates to
nurses' ability to listen to their patients. Before you can listen
attentively to others, it is important to give the individual full
and free attention. This can often be problematic for nurses, as
their minds may be focused on other issues in the environment.
Listening skills involve using body language to convey a
message that you are listening. The nurse should, where
possible, maintain good eye contact and a relaxed, open
posture with a friendly and interested facial expression that
invites the patient to be relaxed.

Encourage the patient to talk by giving an occasional nod of
the head, which demonstrates that you are listening and
understanding. Non-verbal communication can provide a
lot of information about the patient. If an individual becomes
uncomfortable about an aspect of a question, he or she may
avoid eye contact. Outbursts of tears or anger are types of
non-verbal behaviours that communicate feelings such as fear
and anxiety.

There is a wide variety of communication skills that the
nurse can use while interviewing. This includes open and
closed questions. Closed questions, for example, 'Do you have
pain?', can be used to get one- or two-word answers from a
patient; these are particularly useful for confirming specific
information about a patient. Open questions, such as 'How do

you feel?', on the other hand, provide the opportunity to express feelings and invite a response which is much more of the patient's choosing. Although extremely simplistic, as a rule of thumb, 'who', 'what' and 'how' questions tend to elicit more open responses from patients.

Other communication strategies that can be used to elicit information include:

- Facilitation: encourage patients to tell their story.

- Paraphrasing: rephrase what patients have said to you in your own words. This conveys that you're listening and trying to understand them.

- Reflection: repeating back to patients what they have just said to help patients gather their thoughts and elaborate further.

- Clarification: if patients are vague, more explanation may be required.

- Summarising: restate the information given to you by patients.

- Conclusion: final thoughts at the end of the assessment interview.

During the assessment process the physical examination of patients provides the nurse with an opportunity to observe and make judgements about physical signs and symptoms.

Nursing measurements and observations come in many forms, for example taking a pulse or temperature or recording a blood pressure. These are discussed in greater detail in Chapter 4.

One way of organising the information that is required from a nursing assessment is by using a nursing framework. One such framework, the 'activities of living' (ADL), uses a list of patients' activities of living. Through assessment of the 'activities of living', nurses can systematically collect physical and psychosocial information about their patients. The ADL model was devised in Edinburgh during the 1980s by Roper, Logan and Tierney (1985), and it is the most commonly used model in practice in the UK.

The activities of living (ADL) are:

- maintaining a safe environment

- breathing

- eating and drinking

- controlling body temperature

- working and playing

- sleeping

- communication

- eliminating

- personal cleansing

- mobilising

- expressing sexuality

- dying.

Stage 2: Nursing Diagnosis

The second stage of the nursing process involves making a nursing diagnosis. The nurse must translate the information gained during assessment and identify specific nursing problems. Although the word diagnosis is usually associated with the medical profession it should be highlighted that 'diagnosis' is not a concept unique to medicine: car mechanics diagnose mechanical problems, and, in this instance, nurses diagnose nursing problems. Diagnosis is just a general term for identifying a problem. Nursing diagnosis is a critical step in the nursing process. It depends upon an accurate and comprehensive nursing assessment and provides the end-product of the assessment. A clear statement of the patient's problems as ascertained from the nursing assessment is termed as a nursing diagnosis. Nurses can make actual or potential nursing diagnoses. Actual diagnoses are those which have become evident during the assessment. An example of this would be shortness of breath due to respiratory disorder. Conversely, potential diagnoses relate to those which could or will arise as a consequence of the actual diagnoses. For example, an individual who is confined to bed has a greater risk of becoming depressed. Therefore, a potential diagnosis could be the significant risk of depression due to immobility.

A nursing diagnosis is:

• a statement of the patient's problem

• reference to a health problem

• based on objective and subjective data

• a statement of nursing judgement

• a short concise statement

• a condition for which a nurse can independently prescribe care.

Stage 3: Planning Nursing Care

Nursing goals to alleviate or prevent problems identified by assessment can then be determined in the planning stage of the nursing process. This stage involves the prioritisation of patients' problems so that their immediate nursing care needs can be met. There are two stages in the planning stage:

1. Setting goals
2. Identification of actions.

A goal is a statement of what the nurse expects the patient to achieve and is often referred to as an objective. These nursing goals can be short-term or long-term and must be realistic for the patient. Goals serve as the standard by which the nurse can evaluate the effectiveness of nursing action.

The mnemonic checklist MACROS may help the nurse to identify criteria for setting nursing goals:

Measurable or observable
Achievable
Client (or patient)-centred
Realistic
Outcome written
Short.

Action-planning involves planning the care that will ensure that the patient will achieve his or her goals. At this stage, the nurse will specify nursing actions that can be implemented and evaluated. These are the nursing actions, the prescribed interventions that will solve the problem and reach the goal. Another mnemonic, REEPIG, provides criteria that will ensure that planned nursing care is:

Realistic	Are there sufficient resources?
Explicit	Ensure that the planned care is clearly stated.
Evidence-based	Nursing is a research-based profession. The rationale for planned care must be considered.
Prioritise	Nurses should start with the most pressing diagnosis.

| Involvement | Plan of care should not only involve patient. This promotes interprofessional links. |
| Goal-centred | Ensure the care planned meets the set goals. |

Stage 4: Implementation

Implementation comprises the 'doing' phase of the nursing process. It is during this phase that the nurse will put into action the nursing care that is required to address each of the diagnoses and their goals. This stage involves deciding upon appropriate methods to provide nursing care and may involve liaison with other health-care professionals. There are a number of different approaches to the delivery of nursing care that the student nurse should be familiar with. These include:

- task allocation

- patient allocation

- team nursing

- primary nursing

- key worker

- caseload management.

Task allocation is a highly ritualistic system of organising nursing care. Under this system, nurses and support workers are assigned various tasks. For example, one nurse will concentrate on the measurement of vital signs, another nurse focuses on the drug round and so on. Task allocation provides a fragmented approach to nursing care and ensures that the patient will receive aspects of care from a multiplicity of sources. This approach to care provision has been likened to a production line in a factory.

Team nursing is where a designated group of patients is cared for by a team of two or more nurses. These nurses accept full responsibility for the assessment, nursing diagnosis, planning, implementation and evaluation of the patients' care. Each team is headed by a team leader, who must be a registered nurse.

Primary nursing involves a nurse accepting full responsibility and accountability for a patient's care during his or her stay. Primary nursing has been described as a professional patient-centred practice. In its purest form, the implication is that the primary nurse has full responsibility for patients twenty-four hours a day, seven days a week. In reality, a team of nurses provides the care under the direction of the primary nurse, including when the primary nurse is off-duty.

A popular approach to the delivery of care in the fields of mental health and learning difficulties involves the 'key worker'. This relates to one named nurse being responsible for the care of a patient. The key worker will make judgements about when other members of the health-care team are required to be involved with their patient.

In community nursing, caseload management is a very popular way of organising nursing care. It involves a health visitor or district nurse acting as a caseload manager. Caseloads are usually organised on a basis of geographical location or by the GP. Each caseload manager has a team of qualified and health-care support workers to whom specific cases are delegated.

Stage 5: Evaluation

Although this may appear to be the end stage of the nursing process, it is in reality only the end of the beginning and where the process restarts (see Figure 1.1). Evaluation is about reviewing the effectiveness of the nursing care that has been given. It allows the nurse to ascertain whether desired outcomes for the patient have been achieved and it also facilitates the review of the entire nursing process. Evaluation will determine whether a correct nursing diagnosis has been made, whether the assessment was accurate and whether the goals were realistic and achievable. There are several methods that nurses utilise to ensure that appropriate evaluation occurs. These include:

→assessment→diagnosis→planning→implementation→evaluation→

Figure 1.1 Nursing process

• nursing handover

• reflection

• patient satisfaction

• reviewing nursing care plans.

The nursing handover is where a team of nurses hands over information about the nursing care of patients to another group of nurses, usually at the end of a shift. The handover usually involves the nursing care plan as the focus.

At this stage the nursing process may appear a very complex activity that demands a great deal of thought and practice. However, your knowledge and skills will grow and develop as you progress through your nurse training. One such approach involves reflection. Students are recommended to use the following framework to help reflect and learn from their clinical experiences. It involves a staged approach to analysing experiences.

Step 1: Go back to the experience itself and describe exactly what happened. Student should examine how the experience made them feel and how they reacted.

Step 2: Involves concentration on the feelings involved. This may involve positive and negative feelings.

Step 3: The experience should be reworked. In this phase the nurse goes over what happened and thinks about the feelings that the experience generated and links them back to the events.

Step 4: The final stage involves learning from the experience. This starts by asking how you now feel about the experience and how you might have dealt better with the situation. In short, what lessons have been learnt from the experience. Students should learn from both positive and negative experiences.

Reflection should lead the nurse to consider different options in the future, to think more widely. Ultimately, the aim of reflection is to turn experience into learning.

MODELS OF NURSING

Whilst the nursing process provides a framework in which to deliver nursing care, a nursing model provides a structure in which the care is delivered. A model considers the role of the nurse, the needs of the patient and the intended aims of the care provided. A nursing model is comprised of beliefs and values about people, society, health and nursing, and encompasses the physical, psychological and social aspects of health in each of these areas. Ideally, a nursing model is chosen to respond to individual patients' needs. Nursing models are a collection of ideas, knowledge and values about nursing that determines the way nurses work with patients. They help nurses to organise the way they think about their nursing and allow them to practise in an orderly and logical way. Therefore, the primary purpose of models is to help nurses understand nursing from a viewpoint that can directly influence the care they provide. Many nursing models have been created in an attempt to represent the reality of nursing. The activities of living (ADL) model has been devised to help students learn about nursing. The basic premise for a model is a statement about the beliefs and values of a clinical setting that are used as a means of providing effective and evidence-based care; this is usually referred to as the philosophy of the model. With respect to Roper, Logan and Tierney's ADL model it gives Virginia Henderson's definition of nursing as its starting point:

> The unique function of the nurse is to assist the individual, sick or well, in the performance of those activities contributing to health or its recovery (or to a peaceful death) that he [sic] would perform unaided if he had the necessary strength, will or knowledge, and to do this in a way as to help him gain independence as rapidly as possible. (Virginia Henderson, 1966)

Therefore, the belief underpinning the ADL model is that nursing is a helping activity. Using the framework of the ADLs, the nurse aids a patient to gain independence or to die peacefully.

The metaparadigm of nursing

There are four concepts that are found in nursing models or frameworks, which are known as the metaparadigm of nursing. These concepts are:

1. the person
2. the environment
3. health
4. nursing.

All nursing models describe and define these concepts to determine how the care will be provided for the patient. Other concepts may be included within a model to give it a specific focus. Within the ADL model there are several distinctive concepts:

• life span (begins at birth and ends at death)

- dependence/independence continuum

- activities of living (see above)

- preventing activities (e.g. a balanced diet will reduce risk of heart disease)

- individuality in living (each patient is affected by a unique range of factors).

Although concentration has been placed upon the ADL model, there are many other famous nursing models, each with their own specific focus:

- Peplau's model (1952): concept of 'interpersonal relations'

- Orem's model (1980): concept of 'self-care'

- Roy's model (1984): concept of 'adaptation'.

Many clinical areas have attempted to adopt models of nursing to give a more theoretical foundation to their nursing practice. The most common example of how the ADL model is used relates to the assessment and planning of nursing care.

There are several clear benefits from using a model in practice. Models of nursing can be shared by all members of a nursing team and therefore can improve teamwork. Using a nursing model may also direct nursing care by providing a consistent focus to the way in which care is assessed, planned, implemented and evaluated. The ADL model achieves this by providing a comprehensive method of determining nursing needs by means of the activities of living. Additionally, the use of a nursing model will facilitate better communication between members of the nursing team. Through specific documentation or nursing records the progress of the patient can be clearly traced. This, in turn, has led to an improvement in the quality of nursing documentation.

Care pathways

In recent years more attention has been focused upon care pathways for patients. The philosophy behind care pathways is that a planned journey carries less risk than an unplanned journey in the management of an illness and that knowledge of the journey's steps and stages reduces anxiety risks for the patient. The development of pathways for care requires an understanding of the various stages of an illness. For example, patients who have undergone a specific type of surgery will require specialised care at certain points of their hospital stay. This approach to has led to a reduction in the length of hospital stay for some patients.

NURSING IN A MULTIDISCIPLINARY CONTEXT

'Multidisciplinary' is a term used to describe professionals from different disciplines working together. In the health-care setting these professionals work in collaboration to achieve the same goals for the patient. Other terms can be used in place of multidisciplinary, most commonly interprofessional and inter-disciplinary. Examples of professionals involved in patient care include:

doctors	physiotherapists
speech therapists	occupational therapists
dietitians	health visitors
pharmacists	radiographers
district nurses	social workers

Multidisciplinary care can be defined as a group of individuals with different training backgrounds, who share common objectives but who make a different but complementary contribution to care. Working together with other health professionals is part of everyday clinical practice for most nurses. To appreciate the multidisciplinary approach fully, the nurse requires a basic understanding of the role of other health professional groups. Such an understanding will facilitate the key features of this approach: teamwork and collaboration.

FURTHER READING

Grandis, S., Long, G., Glaser, A., and Jackson, P. (eds) (2003) *Foundation Studies for Nursing: Using Enquiry-Based Learning*, London: Palgrave Macmillan.

Hogston, R., and Simpson, P. (eds) (1999) *Foundations of Nursing Practice*, London: Macmillan Press Ltd.

Orem, D. (1991) *Nursing: Concepts of Practice*, 4th edn, St Louis, MO: Mosby.

Roy, C. (1984) *Introduction to Nursing : An Adaptation Model*, 2nd edn, Englewood Cliffs, NJ: Prentice Hall.

2 BIOLOGICAL SCIENCES RELATED TO NURSING

It is essential that all nurses acquire a working knowledge of the human body to be more accountable in practice and become more informed practitioners. The biological science component of nurse education is often found to be the most challenging for nursing students within the university setting. This usually stems from students having had a limited exposure to biological sciences in their school education or to science being taught at a more advanced level at university than school.

While performing fundamental nursing observations, such as taking a temperature, measuring a pulse, recording a blood pressure or testing urine, it is important that nursing students have a thorough understanding of the underlying biological science. It could be argued that there is little point in a nurse recording a temperature if he or she is not aware of the normal temperature or the implications of deviation in temperature, or testing without knowing the normal constituents of urine.

It is only once normal physiological processes are understood that abnormal, that is pathological, processes can be understood and the links between diseases and nursing care can be identified. In many cases it is only once we understand what can go wrong in the body that the rationale behind the treatment interventions becomes clear. Students who struggle to come to terms with biological sciences are, arguably, more likely to have difficulties with the clinically orientated components of nursing courses. Therefore, a good grounding in anatomy and physiology will enable nurses to make well-informed clinical decisions more quickly and accurately.

Material in this chapter will be presented in a standard format, with a brief outline from the characteristics of living matter through to the basic anatomy and physiology of the various systems of the body. The chapter aims to be concise but also to explain the physiology and the necessary basic science in a manner that is easy to understand.

It would be impossible to cover all aspects of anatomy and physiology which are relevant to nurse education in detail within this text. In many instances recommended further reading is provided; it is hoped that this will enable students to clarify any issues that may arise and to supplement their existing knowledge. The recommended texts are written by nurses, specifically, to convey the essential aspects of anatomy and physiology that nursing students require.

BASIC NEEDS OF LIVING MATTER

All living matter is made up of cells. In humans there are hundreds of millions of cells, all working together to make the complete human body. There are several characteristics of living bodies. These are:

- Feeding: relates to the intake of raw materials (food) to maintain life processes.

- Respiration: refers to the processes by which energy is produced to maintain life processes. In humans this relates to breathing (external respiration) and the breakdown of food (internal respiration) inside the cells of the body.

- Growth: includes the repair of body parts (e.g. wound repair after surgery).

- Excretion: the removal of waste products from the body. These waste products include sweat from the skin and urine from the kidneys.

- Movement: the ability to change position.

- Sensitivity: the processes concerned with monitoring, detecting and responding to changes in the environment inside and outside the body. This relates to the concept of homeostasis (see below).

- Reproduction: all living matter needs to reproduce its own kind. This is the process by which continuation of the species occurs.

Nurses should be able to relate their knowledge of biological sciences to the care of patients. It is useful at this stage to define a few terms commonly used in the study of biological science.

- physiology: the study of the normal function of the human body

- anatomy: the study of the structure of the body

- pathology: the study of abnormal anatomy

- pathophysiology: the study of abnormal body functions.

As well as understanding the fundamentals of anatomy and physiology, an elementary knowledge of chemistry and physics will enable nurses to better understand medical and nursing procedures.

- chemistry: the study of the composition of matter and the reaction between various types of matter

- physics: the study of the behaviour and characteristics of matter (e.g. in the measurement of blood pressure or recording of blood gases).

It is anticipated (hoped) that potential student nurses have had some background in physical sciences and as such these will be addressed in relation to specific nursing activities in this text.

HOMEOSTASIS

Within the study of anatomy and physiology is the central concept of homeostasis (from the Greek 'staying the same'). Homeostasis refers to the automatic, self-regulatory processes that are necessary to maintain the 'normal' state of the body's environment. Homeostasis represents the processes necessary for the maintenance of conditions under which the body can function at its best. The concept of homeostasis is fundamental to an understanding of human biology, as homeostasis ensures the basic necessities of health. Illness commonly results in deviations from homeostasis. The process of homeostasis is self-regulating and each body system that is examined in this section is involved in this regulation.

As the aim of homeostasis is to maintain a constant internal environment for cells of the body to survive and function, any alteration of temperature, acid-base (pH) and electrolyte balance may result in the rapid death of cells. Homeostasis regulates blood levels of oxygen, carbon dioxide, electrolytes, glucose and hormones. As such, homeostasis controls the function of many body systems, including respiratory and urinary, and is instrumental in regulating body temperature and blood pressure. The maintenance of homeostasis is therefore the most important physiological function of the body.

How does homeostasis work?

Homeostasis is a dynamic system that allows the body to respond to changing conditions. Most homeostatic control mechanisms are maintained on the principle of negative feedback. The components of a negative feedback are threefold: a detector, an effector and a control area. The detector, or monitor, senses a change in the internal environment of the body; the effector institutes a change in order to return the internal environment to homeostasis; and the control area determines what the normal physiological situation should be by decreasing the action of the effector once homeostasis has been achieved.

Homeostasis keeps a number of bodily functions within a reasonably narrow range through its ability to detect movement beyond or outside these normal parameters and make the appropriate corrections. One good example of homeostasis is the regulation of blood pressure. The control centre is the hypothalamus, in the brain, and changes in blood pressure are detected by a system of pressure receptors (baroreceptors) in the cardiovascular system; the effector is a combination of the action of the heart and blood vessels. The baroreceptors respond to stretch and as the blood pressure increases in the cardiovascular system they are stretched and send signals to the control centre in the hypothalamus that the pressure is increasing in the system. In response the hypothalamus sends signals to the cardiovascular system through nerves and hormones, which result in a lower blood pressure. Therefore, the combined action of the hormonal system and nerves control blood pressure.

Maintaining homeostasis is undoubtedly the most important physiological function of the body. A significant part of the nursing role is to compensate for disturbances in homeostasis. Nurses are often involved in helping sick individuals to overcome the effects of illness or trauma, which can leave the body in homeostatic imbalance.

The remainder of this chapter provides an introduction to the basic anatomy and physiology of the systems of the body.

Levels of organisation and homeostasis

There is a clear logic to the way that the human body is organised anatomically and physiologically. All living matter is composed of the basic units of life known as cells. Groups of cells similar in appearance, function and origin combine together to form tissues. Different tissues then interact with each other to form organs. Finally, groups of organs interact to form body systems. Consequently, four levels of organisation exist in the human body: cells, tissues, organs and systems.

CELLS

Cells are the basic building blocks in humans. Most human cells are microscopic, with the average size ranging from 15 to 30 micrometres (micrometre = one thousandth of a millimetre) in diameter. Cellular anatomy varies to allow cells to perform different functions and maintain body homeostasis. The majority of human cells have certain features in common.

Cytology is the term used to describe the study of cells (*'cyt'* = cell, *'-logy'* = study).

Cells that make up a particular tissue are themselves composed of smaller functional units called cell organelles. These organelles can be thought of as the 'organs' of the cell and include:

- cell (plasma) membrane

- endoplasmic reticulum (smooth and rough)

- golgi complex

- lysosomes

- mitochondria

- nucleus.

Cell (plasma) membrane

The cell or plasma membrane plays an important role by holding the contents of the cell together and regulating the control of fluids, electrolytes, nutrients and waste products in and out the cell. This thin membrane is described as semi- or selectively permeable and it surrounds the outside and as such marks the boundary of the cell. The membrane separates the intracellular ('intra' = inside) from extracellular ('extra' = outside) environment and is composed of protein and a substance called phospholipids. Some of the proteins in the membrane act as receptor sites and these allow the cell to recognise chemical messages from other cells or from endocrine glands.

Transport across the plasma membrane
Movement of substances across the cell membrane can take place by several processes:

- osmosis

- simple diffusion

- facilitated diffusion

- active transport.

Osmosis relates to the movement of water or solvent chemicals from a higher to lower concentration via a selectively permeable membrane.

Simple diffusion relates to the net movement of chemicals from regions of high concentration to regions of a lower concentration, until they are evenly distributed. An example of diffusion in the body can be seen in the movement of oxygen from the lungs into blood; from blood, oxygen diffuses into tissue fluid and from tissue fluid into cells. No energy is required for diffusion.

Facilitated diffusion can only take place when the concentration of the substance outside the cell is greater than the concentration inside the cell. The presence of protein carriers in the plasma membrane allows for the passage of substances through protein channels. Some cells accumulate nutrients such as carbohydrates (glucose molecules) in this manner.

Another process by which substances can be accumulated or

expelled from the cell is active transport. Energy is required for this process. This energy-release process is termed oxidative phosphorylation, during which adenosine diphosphate (ADP) is converted to adenosine triphosphate (ATP) with the release of energy. Oxygen is essential to facilitate this process.

There are several factors which can influence the transport of substances across cell membranes. These include:

• Chemical size (larger molecules are slower than smaller ones)

• Chemical solubility (oil soluble > water soluble due to phospholipids in membrane)

• Chemical charge of substance (uncharged are more likely to be transported)

• Temperature (a higher temperature increases the movement of chemicals).

The remaining organelles of the cell have specific roles to play in the maintainance of homeostasis in the human cell. It is important to understand that although each organelle is considered individually, they all work interdependently.

Endoplasmic reticulum

Endoplasmic reticulum is a membrane system of channels distributed throughout the cytoplasm of a cell. The most basic function of endoplasmic is to move materials around the cell. In a sense endoplasmic reticulum can be thought of as a transport network for the cell, delivering raw materials to various destinations. Additionally, endoplasmic reticulum provides support for the overall shape and structure of the cell.

Rough endoplasmic reticulum/ribosomes

Rough, or granular, endoplasmic reticulum has a distinctive appearance as it is studded with ribosomes on its outer surface. Ribosomes are small dark-staining organelles which receive genetic instructions form deoxyribonucleic acid (DNA) in the nucleus of the cell. They use this information to string together long chains of amino acids, the building blocks of proteins, to assemble protein molecules. Ribosomes are therefore the site of protein synthesis in the cell and can be thought of as 'protein factories'. Rough endoplasmic reticulum is extremely important within the cell as it contributes directly to the maintenance of intracellular (within cell) homeostasis.

Golgi complex

The golgi complex, also termed golgi body or apparatus, is an arrangement of membranes which are responsible for the export of products from the cell. Golgi is found in all human cells except red blood cells. Products of the endoplasmic reticulum are transported to the golgi complex, where modifications take place. The principal homeostatic role of the golgi complex is processing and delivering chemicals to various parts of the cell. In addition, secretory products are packaged in this region prior to release. One example of this function can be seen in the cells of the digestive system which secrete digestive enzymes that aid the digestive process.

Lysosomes

Lysosomes originate from the golgi complex. They have a thicker membrane than other organelles as they contain many digestive enzymes, such as lysozyme. This thicker membrane is required to separate the enzymes from the rest of the cell parts as enzymes are capable of breaking down all the chemical components of the cell. Enzymes are protein catalysts that accelerate chemical reactions but do not actually take part in the reaction and therefore remain unchanged by it. Enzymes, like most proteins, are produced in the rough endoplasmic reticulum. These are then transported to the golgi complex. Lysosomes are found in most human cells, especially very active cells, such as liver cells.

Cystol

Cystol is the fluid found in the cytoplasm of a cell. It contains water and larger molecules: in combination these are referred to as a colloid. The cellular organelles are suspended with cystol.

Mitochondria

Mitochondria give cells the ability to produce energy and to fuel physiological processes. The size, shape and number of mitochondria vary from cell to cell depending upon their level of activity. The basic structure involves a double-membraned organelle. The enfolded inner membrane provides a large surface area responsible for the generation of energy within the cell. Cells that are very active, such as those in the liver, have many mitochondria in their cytoplasm, whereas cells that require less energy, such as in the skin, have far fewer.

Nucleus

The nucleus of a cell is usually located in the centre within the cytoplasm. It is surrounded by a separate membrane, the nuclear membrane. Located within the nucleus of human cells are chromosomes. Each cell contains 46 chromosome bodies, arranged in 23 pairs; these chromosomes contain genes made of DNA, which provide the genetic information responsible for making and controlling the cell.

Chromosomes

The chromosomes are composed of structural proteins and acid DNA. Genes contain the genetic information required to create a cell.

Specialised cells

During growth and development, cells have the ability to carry out various functions. The process of cell specialisation is termed 'differentiation'. Specialised cells are required to form the different types of tissues and organs throughout the body.

Cell reproduction

There are two distinct types of cell division: mitosis and meiosis. In the human body cell division take place by mitosis, during which a parent cell containing 46 chromosomes divides into two daughter cells, each of which consists of 46 chromosomes. Cell produced by this type of division are called somatic cells.

There are several phases in mitosis:

- prophase

- metaphase

- anaphase

- telophase

- formation of daughter cells.

Meiosis
Meiosis is referred to as 'reduction division' as the resultant daughter cells only have 23 chromosomes. Meiosis is only used in the production of gametes, that is sperm and ova.

TISSUES

As cells become more specialised they form into groups called tissues. A simple definition of a tissue is a group of cells similar in appearance, origin and function. In the human body there are four main types of tissue:

• epithelial

• connective

• muscular

• nervous.

Epithelial describes any type of tissue that lines or covers another structure. The internal and external surfaces throughout the body are lined with epithelial tissue.

The two main types of epithelium are simple and stratified. Simple epithelium is composed of a single layer of cells attached to a basement membrane. Simple epithelium is usually very delicate and is found in regions of the body where there is little wear and tear. Different forms of epithelial tissue are described according to their shape. These include:

• squamous: flat, smooth surface (e.g. lining of blood vessels)

• cuboidal: cube-shaped, found in endocrine glands

• columnar: column-shaped, found in gastrointestinal tract.

The presence of microscopic hair-like processes projecting from the surface of simple columnar epithelial cells can be seen in the respiratory tract; these projections are called cilia. The ciliated cells help to waft mucus from the smaller airways to the trachea.

Stratified epithelium

Stratified epithelium is made up of many layers of cells, some of which are not in direct contact with the basement membrane. The presence of several layers of cells is shown in Figure 2.1. There are different types of stratified epithelium, which comprise layers of cells. For example, stratified squamous epithelium consists of several layers of flat cells. Usually stratified epithelium is only found in areas of the body which are subjected to a high degree of wear and tear. One example of this is in the mouth, where a lining of stratified squamous epithelium help deal with the presence of foodstuff during chewing. Some types of stratified epithelium which are subjected to the greatest wear and tear, such as skin, are keratinised. Keratin is a protein that provides resistance to wear and tear and is waterproof.

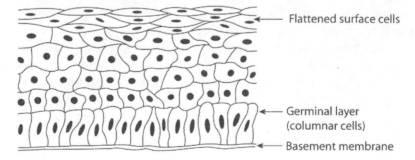

Figure 2.1 Stratified epithelium

Transitional cells

Transitional epithelium is similar to stratified epithelium. However, in transitional cells the surface cells are designed to stretch and appear pear-shaped as opposed to being flattened. This type of epithelium is found lining organs which must be able to expand (e.g. the urinary bladder).

Glands

Glands develop from epithelial tissues in the human body. They have the ability to make specific secretions. For example, the gastric glands in the stomach produce hydrochloric acid, which is found in gastric juice.

Connective Tissue

Connective tissue supports and binds together tissues. Examples of connective tissue include tendons and ligaments.

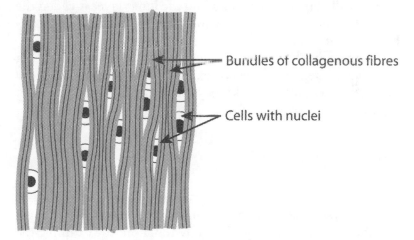

Figure 2.2 Dense connective tissue

The study of tissues is known as histology. Histology provides an important branch of medicine because it can be used to detect diseased tissue. Nurses deal with many connective tissue disorders including systemic lupus erythematosus and scleroderma.

ORGANS

Groups of tissues interact to produce larger structures known as organs. An example of an organ which relates to digestion is the stomach. The stomach is an organ which is composed of several types of tissue, including smooth muscle tissue, endothelial tissue, glandular tissue and nervous tissue. Organs are described as being either tubular or compact. Tubular organs have common features:

• A space called the lumen.

• Tubular structure: outer epithelial layer; middle layer containing muscle; and inner endothelial layer.

The heart is an example of a tubular organ in the human body. The outer layer is called the pericardium, the middle layer is called the myocardium and the inner layer is called the endocardium. Within the lumen of the heart are four chambers, the atria and ventricles.

Compact organs have no lumen. They are composed of a superficial layer called the cortex and a deeper layer called the medulla. The liver and kidneys are examples of compact organs in the human body.

BODY SYSTEMS

Groups of organs interact to form the next level of organisation, the system. An organ system is a group of organs that act together to perform a specific body function, for example the digestive system digests, absorbs and processes food taken in as nutrients. Systems of the body work with each other in a coordinated manner to maintain the functions of the body. These systems are the subject of the remainder of this section. Examples of systems of the human body are given in Table 2.1.

Table 2.1 Systems of the body

Skeletal system	provides a framework which gives support and protection to tissues and allows movement.
Muscular system	effects movement of the body as a whole.
Nervous system	creates an awareness of the environment.
Circulatory system	known as the internal transport system of the body.
Respiratory system	allows exchange of gases between environment and body.
Lymphatic system	consists of lymphatic drainage vessels and other structures that contain lymphatic tissue
Integumentary system	consists of the skin and its accessory structures.
Digestive system	concerned with digestion and absorption of food.
Urinary system	the main excretory system of the body.
Reproductive system	responsible for survival of the species.

Skeletal System

The skeletal and muscular systems enable us to maintain a posture against gravity and to move in a co-ordinated way. Failure to maintain the flexibility of joints, strong bones and contraction of appropriate muscles rapidly induces inadequate mobilisation. Nurses should be aware that lack of mobility can lead to dependency on other people, in order to perform the most basic activities of daily living.

The nervous system

The nervous system enables us to monitor and maintain a
constant internal environment as well as monitor and respond
to an external environment. It consists of the Central Nervous
System (CNS), which includes the brain and spinal cord,
which in turn is connected to other parts of the body via
the Peripheral Nervous System (PNS).

Central Nervous System
The brain and the spinal cord are surrounded by bone (skull
and vertebrae) and are insulated by fluid and tissue. The brain
is composed of three parts:

1. **Cerebrum** is the largest part of the brain and is
   described as the 'seat of consciousness'. It includes the
   cerebral hemispheres, which are separated by the
   corpus callosum. In humans, the cerebrum co-
   ordinates sensory and motor functions, as well as
   governing intelligence and reasoning, learning and
   memory.
2. **Cerebellum** is the second largest part of the brain and is
   part of the unconscious brain. It functions for muscle
   co-ordination; maintains normal muscle tone and
   posture; and controls balance.
3. **Medulla** and brainstem (including the midbrain and
   pons) are also part of the unconscious brain. The
   medulla is closest to the spinal cord and is involved
   with regulation of breathing, blood pressure and heart
   rate, and controls swallowing, sneezing, coughing and
   vomiting.

The spinal cord is the major pathway connecting the brain
and Peripheral Nervous System to the rest of the body. It is
about 45cm long in men and 43cm long in women. The length
of the spinal cord is much shorter than the length of the bony
spinal column.

Peripheral Nervous System

There are two main components of the peripheral nervous system (PNS):

1. Sensory (afferent) pathways provide input from the body into the CNS.
2. Motor (efferent) pathways carry signals to muscles and glands.

The motor nervous system comprises the somatic nervous system, which innervates the muscular system resulting in the contraction and relaxation of muscles, and the autonomic nervous system (ANS), which controls smooth muscle in internal organs. The ANS is in turn divided into the sympathetic nervous system (involved in the fight-or-flight response) and the parasympathetic nervous system (involved in relaxation). These two systems operate automatically.

Nervous tissue

There are two main cell types:

1. Neurones – transmit nerve messages
2. Glial cells – are in direct contact with neurones and often surround them.

The neurone is the functional unit of the nervous system and we have about 100 billion in our brain alone. Any neurone can be divided up into cell body and extensions (neurites: dentrites and axons). Dentrites receive information from another cell and transmit the message to the cell body. The axon conducts messages away from the cell. Some axons are wrapped by specialised glial cells (mylinated axons), which help to increase the speed at which the impulses are conducted. Axons of neurones are grouped together to form nerve fibres. Nerves are distinct peripheral extensions of the CNS, thirty-one pairs leave the spinal cord (spinal nerves) and twelve pairs leave the brain (cranial nerves).

The nerve message

Information from one neurone flows to another neurone across a synapse (a small gap separating neurones). For communication between neurones to occur, an electrical impulse must travel down an axon, away from the cell body, to the synaptic terminal. This 'impulse' is called an Action Potential and it is the way the neurone responds to excitatory stimulation.

Communication of information between neurones is accomplished by movement of chemicals across the synapse. Chemicals, called neurotransmitters, are released from one neurone where they may be accepted by the next neurone at a specialised site called a receptor. The action that follows activation of a receptor site may be either depolarisation (an excitatory postsynaptic potential) or hyperpolarisation (an inhibitory postsynaptic potential). A depolarisation makes it more likely that an Action Potential will fire; a hyperpolarisation makes it less likely that an Action Potential will fire.

The circulatory system

In order to remain alive, cells require a continuous supply of oxygen and nutrients for their metabolism. The cardiovascular system provides a transport system for the supply and removal of materials to and from tissue cells; it consists of the heart, blood and blood vessels. The heart works as a circulatory pump and the blood vessels work as a closed transporting system, which delivers blood to all parts of the body. Blood is a tissue which has several functions in the human body, including transport of gases (oxygen and carbon dioxide), defence against infection, clotting, and distribution of heat and transport of nutrients.

The heart

The heart is a hollow, muscular pump, which is located between the lungs and extends to the left-hand side of the thoracic cavity. The heart is protected from physical trauma

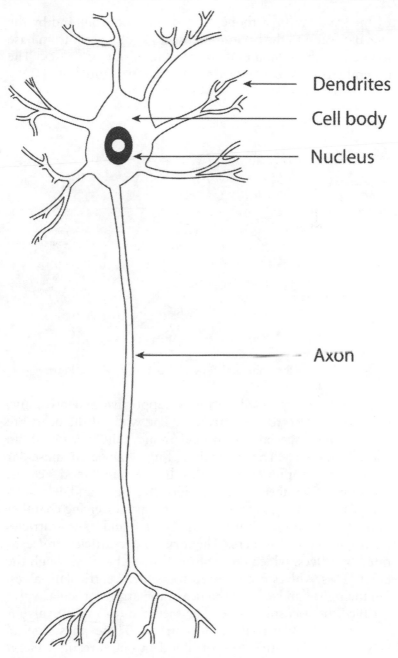

Dendrites

Cell body

Nucleus

Axon

Figure 2.3 Structure of a neurone

by the sternum (breastbone) and ribs to the front and by the spinal column to the back. It measures about 12cm from base to apex, is about 9cm in diameter and about 6cm thick. The general structure of the heart is shown in Figure 2.4.

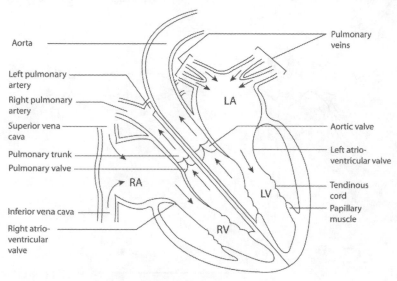

Figure 2.4 Structure and flow of blood through the heart

The heart is enclosed within a supportive and protective membrane called the pericardium. The walls of the heart are composed of specialised muscle tissue called myocardium (cardiac muscle). The heart is a four-chambered muscular pump that continuously pumps blood into blood vessels. The upper chamber on each side, the right and left atria (singular = atrium), is smaller and acts as a receiving chamber into which blood flows via veins. The left and right ventricles form the lower chambers. The atria and ventricles are separated by valves, which control the flow of blood through the heart. These valves are referred to as atrioventricular valves. On the right-hand side of the heart, the atrioventricular valve is called the tricuspid valve. The bicuspid (or mitral) valve is between the left atrium and ventricle. These physiological valves only allow the flow of blood in one direction. Heart valves are attached to the ventricular walls by tendons called chordae tendinea; these are connected to the heart by specialised muscle tissue called papillary muscles. The left- and right-hand side of the heart are separated by the cardiac septum. This means that blood from the right-hand side of the heart cannot mix with blood from the left-hand side and vice versa.

Functionally the heart can be thought of as two pumps:

1. Left side of heart: pumps blood to body (systemic circulation).
2 Right side of heart: pumps blood to lungs (pulmonary circulation).

The myocardium has specialised cardiac cells that are linked by branches; this allows them to contract simultaneously, acting as a single unit or functional syncytium. The impulse to contract arises through spontaneous depolarisation in an area of specialised tissue called the sinoatrial (SA) node, the pacemaker of the heart. From the SA node an impulse spreads across both atria stimulating their contraction. The atrioventricular valve (AV) collects the impulse from the atria and passes it on to the atrioventricular bundle in the cardiac septum. In the cardiac septum the atrioventricular bundle divides into two, the right and left bundle branches, which carry the impulses to the respective ventricles. The impulse innervates the ventricular myocardial muscles via the small Purkinje fibres.

The heart beats approximately eighty times each minute. The rate varies with age, illness, emotion and exercise. The cardiac cycle is the period between the end of one heartbeat to the end of the next. Each beat of the cycle lasts about 0.8 seconds. The term for contraction is systole and the term for relaxation is diastole.

● Systole (ventricular contraction) relates to blood being pushed out of the heart

● Diastole (ventricular relaxation) is the refilling phase of the heart.

Cardiac output is the volume of blood pumped out of a single ventricle in one minute. The formula for cardiac output is the heart rate multiplied by stroke volume. Where:

Heat rate = the number of times the heart beats per minute.
Stroke volume = the amount of blood pumped out of the heart per cardiac contraction.

At rest a normal stroke volume is 70ml; if the heart rate is 70 beats a minute this would give a cardiac output of 4900ml. During vigorous exercise cardiac output can be greater than 30 litres per minute!

Control of the heart
The heart is innervated by the autonomic nervous system, which maintains heart rate at an average level. The sympathetic component of the autonomic nervous system increases heart rate, whereas the parasympathetic component, via the vagus nerve (tenth crainial nerve), slows the heart down and causes decreased power of contraction by conveying impulses to the SA node. The sympathetic nerves speed the heart rate and increase the force of contraction. This control of heart rate is co-ordinated by the cardiac centre in the medulla oblongata in the brain. The heart rate is also controlled reflexly by two sets of receptors:

- Baroreceptor: sensitive to changes in blood pressure

- Chemoreceptors: sensitive to the amount of oxygen and CO_2 in blood.

Baroreceptors are found in the arch of the aorta and in the carotid artery provide an example of a homeostatic mechanism which controls blood-pressure regulation by negative feedback. If blood pressure increases, less sympathetic stimulation and more parasympathetic stimulation is observed and heart rate slows down, reducing the blood pressure. Chemoreceptors are sensitive to high levels of carbon dioxide and to low levels of oxygen. Impulses are conveyed to the cardiac centre, in the medulla oblongata, and heart rate is increased, giving an increased oxygenated blood to the tissues.

The influence of heart rate upon blood pressure is given further attention with relation to measurement of clinical observations in Chapter 4.

The blood vessels

Blood circulates through a closed system of blood vessels throughout the body. The main types of blood vessel in the human body are arteries, capillaries and veins. Blood flows away from the heart in arteries that divide into smaller arterioles and then into capillaries. The blood then flows back to the heart via the venous system. The system that supplies blood to the body is referred to as the arterial system and that which returns blood to the heart is the venous system.

Arteries are thick-walled vessels that carry blood away from the heart. With one exception, the pulmonary arteries, they are involved in the transport of oxygenated blood. The exception is the pulmonary artery, which carries deoxygenated blood to the lungs from the right-hand side of the heart to the lungs. Arteries have thick walls because they carry blood at a fairly high pressure. Blood flows along arteries due to the pumping effect of the heart generating a blood pressure. Because the arteries carry blood directly from the heart, a pulse can be felt every time the heart contracts. Measurement of pulse rate is examined in Chapter 4.

All arteries walls have three layers (see Figure 2.5):

● tunica externa (adventitia): the outer coat

● tunica media: the middle coat

● tunica interna (intima): the inner coat.

The space in the middle of any blood vessel is referred to as the lumen. All of the systemic arteries in the body branch from the main artery, the aorta. Other main arteries include the hepatic artery to the liver and the renal artery to the kidneys. Small arteries divide into smaller vessels called arterioles. These have a similar structure to arteries, but the interna and media are thinner and the externa is thicker than in arteries. Arterioles are important in the regulation of blood pressure in the body. Constriction of an arteriole will narrow the lumen of the arterial system; this in turn will increase resistance to blood flow. This resistance to blood flow is termed peripheral resistance and will result in an increase in blood pressure. Conversely, if peripheral resistance is lowered due to dilation of arterioles (vasodilation), blood pressure will be lowered. The other factor which influences blood pressure relates to the volume of blood pumped from the heart (cardiac volume). Therefore, blood pressure can be simply defined as peripheral resistance multiplied by cardiac volume. This is further examined in Chapter 4 (see section on measurement of blood pressure).

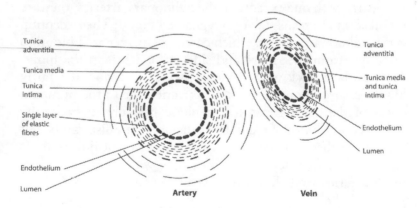

Figure 2.5 Structure of arteries and veins

Capillaries form a network between arterioles and venules (little veins). They are the smallest blood vessels and receive blood from arterioles. Capillaries are the only part of the circulatory system where there is exchange of materials between the blood and tissues; all other vessels are too thick to allow this. Capillaries can facilitate exchanges as they are only one squamous cell thick. Overall, the capillaries form a massive surface between the blood and the tissues. The total area of capillary wall in an adult is approximately 6000 square metres.

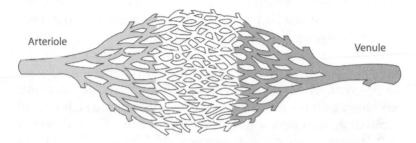

Arteriole

Venule

Figure 2.6 Capillary network

Structure of veins

A vein is defined as any vessel that carries blood towards the heart. Veins and venules have the same three-layered structure as arteries, with a central lumen, tunica externa, tunica media and tunica interna. The middle layer of veins is thinner than that of arteries, due to a lower pressure in the venous system. Unlike arteries, veins have physiological valves within their lumen to prevent the backflow of blood.

Pulmonary veins carry oxygenated blood to the lungs and systemic veins carry deoxygenated blood. The pressure of blood within the venous circulation is low and provides little force to circulate blood.

Veins are adapted with thin walls, larger diameter lumens and valves to aid the return of blood to the heart. In fact, the thin walls and large lumen means that about two-thirds of total blood volume is found within the venous system at any time, which is why veins are referred to as blood reservoirs. Venous return is also aided by the contraction of adjacent skeletal muscles. When a muscle contracts, veins within the muscle are squeezed and as a result the lumen of the vein is reduced in size, allowing the blood to flow towards the heart.

Mechanisms of circulation and issues surrounding blood

pressure and pulse measurement are discussed in Chapter 4 on clinical observations.

Blood

Blood is a very complex fluid. It is classified as connective tissue as it contains both cells and plasma. It forms about 5 per cent of body weight, so the average human being contains three to four litres. Cells account for approximately 45 per cent of blood volume and plasma accounts for the remaining 55 per cent. The blood cells carry out a variety of functions: red blood cells transport gases whilst white blood cells defend the body against invasion by micro-organisms. Thrombocytes, or platelets, consist of fragments of larger cells and are principally concerned with the formation of blood clots following injury.

The main functions of blood are the following:

- to carry oxygen to the tissues (via oxyhaemoglobin)

- to carry nutrients to the tissue

- to carry water to the tissues

- to carry away waste products to organs

- to fight bacterial infections (white blood cells)

- to provide materials for glands to make their secretions

- to distribute secretions (e.g. hormones)

- to distribute heat around the body

- to arrest haemorrhage via the clotting process.

Plasma

Plasma is a clear, straw-coloured, watery fluid. It is made up of 90 per cent water and a mix of various substances in solution, including plasma proteins (e.g. albumin, fibrinogen and globulin), mineral salts (e.g. chlorides and phosphates), foodstuffs, regulatory chemical (e.g. enzymes and hormones), gases in solution (e.g. oxygen, carbon dioxide and nitrogen) and waste products from tissues (e.g. urea and creatinine).

Blood cells
There are three types of blood cell:

- red blood cells (erythrocytes)

- white blood cells (leucocytes)

- platelets (thrombocytes).

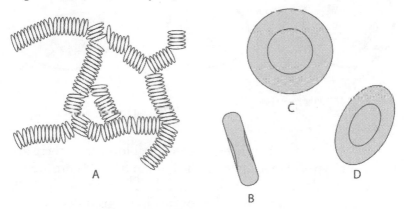

Figure 2.7 Red blood cells

Red blood cells are minute biconcave disc-shaped bodies. The main function of red blood cells is to carry oxygen from the lungs to tissues and cells. They have an average lifespan of 120 days and are very numerous in the human body, numbering in the region of 5 million per cubic millilitre of blood. To understand how small they are, each red blood cell has a diameter of only 7.2 micrometres (one micrometre = a thousandth of a millimetre). The haematocrit is the percentage of blood that is composed of red blood cells and can be used as a clinical indicator of anaemia.

Erythrocytes have no nucleus, which increases their oxygen-carrying capacity, but they do contain a special protein known as haemoglobin.

Haemoglobin is a protein pigment which is yellow in colour, although the massed effect of the numerous cells gives blood its distinctive red colour. It is haemoglobin that actually carries oxygen in red blood cells; one haemoglobin molecule can form a loose bond with four oxygen molecules. Each haemoglobin molecule is based upon four atoms of iron. Without iron, haemoglobin cannot be synthesised, and so this underlines the importance of iron in the diet.

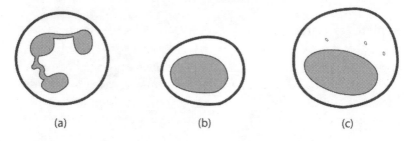

(a)   (b)   (c)

Figure 2.8 White blood cells

Leucocyte is the general term for white blood cells; there are two main types of leucocytes in the human body. There are far less white cells in the body than red cells, approximately 7000 per cubic millimetre. Some leucocytes have granules in their cytoplasm and are classified as granulocytes, others have a clear cytoplasm and as such are called agranulocytes.

Ranulocytes are further classified, according to their staining properties, into neutrophils, eosinophils and basophils.

Neutrophils are the most common type of granular leucocytes. They compose 70 per cent of white cells in the blood. The granules in their cytoplasm contain a variety of enzymes which are able to digest small particles of cell debris and bacteria. This process of ingestion is called phagocytosis, and neutrophils can be known as phagocytes.

Phagocytosis is a process whereby cells ingest and digest material that the immune system has identified for destruction.

If infection is present in the body the number of neutrophils will greatly increase to combat the causative micro-organisms, a process known as neutrophil leucocytosis.

Eosinophils are slightly larger than neutrophils. Normally, 2–4 per cent of the leucocytes found in blood are eosinophils. Eosinophils help the body fight infections and are also able to chemically neutralise histamines, which are involved in allergic response. An increase in their number is seen in allergic conditions (e.g. asthma).

Basophils are extremely uncommon in blood and compose less than 0.5 per cent of white cells. The granules in basophils contain histamine and heparin. Although the precise function of basophils remains unclear, they are known to play an important part in allergic reactions, such as hayfever.

Lymphocytes make up 20 per cent of the total white-cell count. They are produced in lymph nodes and are concerned with the production of antibodies. An increase in the number of lymphocytes is known as lymphocytosis; this occurs when more antibodies are produced to counter infection. Monocytes are the largest white blood cells. They make up 5 per cent of the total white-cell count. Monocytes are referred to as macrophages. If they encounter any bacteria they will destroy them. The number of monocytes is most likely to increase during a chronic bacterial infection.

Thrombocytes, or platelets, are fragments of larger white cells that circulate in the blood. They play an important role in the clotting of blood. If there is a deficiency of thrombocytes then blood clotting will be impaired, resulting in haemorrhage and bruising. A lack of thrombocytes in the body is known as thrombocytopenia.

Haemostasis

The process by which blood loss from the body is prevented following trauma (i.e. a cut) is called haemostasis and involves three stages which are closely related. Bleeding, or haemorrhage, can occur for any type of blood vessel and the stages of haemostasis can be summarised as follows:

- Vascular spasm – the lumen of the damaged blood vessel narrows to slow down the loss of blood.

- A platelet plug forms to stop the flow of blood from the damaged vessel.

- A fibrin clot forms to seal the damaged vessel.

The clotting process is referred to as the coagulation cascade and is a very complex process which involves many factors. The end point of the process is the formation of an insoluble clot from soluble fibrinogen and this process is initiated by the formation of thrombin. The extrinsic and intrinsic systems stimulate the formation of thrombin by the formation of prothrombin activator. Prothrombin is essential for all blood clotting throughout the body and is therefore continually synthesised in the liver. Vitamin K is required for the formation of prothrombin and fibrinogen. Patients with liver disease or Vitamin K deficiency may therefore suffer from bleeding disorders. A more comprehensive overview of haemostasis is provided in the recommend texts.

The respiratory system

All living cells require a constant supply of oxygen to carry out their metabolism and to help maintain homeostasis. During inspiration humans breathe air into paired lungs via the nose and mouth. Oxygen, which is present in atmospheric air, is taken into the lungs, where it can be extracted for utilisation in the body. Simultaneously carbon dioxide and waste products are given up for release. Maintaining an adequate supply of oxygen is essential for the metabolic homeostasis of cells and tissues.

Tissue oxygenation occurs in four stages:

1. Oxygen is taken up from atmospheric air by blood.
2. Oxygen is carried by the blood.

3. Tissues receive adequate perfusion with blood.

4. Oxygen passes from blood to cells.

Once within the cell oxygen can be utilised (e.g. oxidative phosphorylation). If carbon-dioxide levels in the body become excessive these can be potentially harmful. Therefore, carbon dioxide, produced in the tissues, is excreted.

The following are the main structures of the respiratory system; they can also be seen in Figure 2.9.

• nose

• pharynx

• larynx

• trachea

• bronchi

• bronchioles

• alveolar ducts and alveoli

• lungs.

General terms used in relation to the respiratory system:

• respiration: production of energy by cells

• internal respiration: reactions taking place within cells that consume oxygen and release carbon dioxide

• external respiration: processes occurring within the lungs, taking up oxygen from atmospheric air and releasing carbon dioxide into it

- inspiration: the process of breathing in

- expiration: the process of breathing out

- hypoxia: a shortage of oxygen at the level of tissues.

Nose
Humans breathe air into paired lungs through the nose and mouth during inspiration. As air passes through the nasal passage it is warmed, which prevents the lower airways being chilled. The cavity of the nose is lined throughout with a ciliated mucous membrane, which is extremely vascular. The mucus moistens the air and filters it to remove dust and other foreign particles. Receptors for the sense of smell are located in the olfactory epithelium, which is in the roof of the nasal cavity. Humans can distinguish up to 4000 different odours.

Pharynx
The pharynx has two components: the oropharynx forms the throat, and the nasopharynx is an extension of the throat up to the nasal cavities. The opening into the airways from the oropharynx is called the glottis, which is closed off during swallowing by a small flap called the epiglottis (see Figure 2.9). If this fails to work, food may enter the airway, described as going down the 'wrong way', and may lead to choking.

Larynx
After the glottis, the inspired air enters the larynx, a structure of cartilage and ligaments that forms the Adam's apple. As the larynx contains the vocal cords or folds, it is referred to as the 'voicebox'. The vocal cords are composed of elastic ligaments that can be tightened or relaxed. Sound is produced by air passing across these cords, causing them to vibrate.

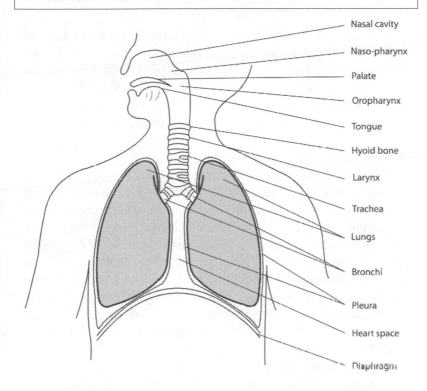

Nasal cavity

Naso-pharynx

Palate

Oropharynx

Tongue

Hyoid bone

Larynx

Trachea

Lungs

Bronchi

Pleura

Heart space

Diaphragm

Figure 2.9 The respiratory tract

Trachea

The trachea, or windpipe, begins below the larynx and runs down the front of the neck into the chest and on average it is 10cm long. It is vital to ensure that the trachea is open at all times as it is the only way that air can reach the lungs. The walls of the trachea are strengthened by 16–20 C-shaped rings of cartilage, which prevent it collapsing. The trachea divides into two branches known as the left and right primary bronchus, one entering each lung (see Figure 2.9).

Bronchi

Each primary bronchus divides into a secondary bronchi, referred to as lobar bronchi, because one enters each lobe of the lung. Each of these then divides into named branches, one for each broncho-pulmonary segment. The smallest bronchi are called bronchioles. They have no cartilage but are composed of muscular, fibrous and elastic tissue lined with cuboidal epithelium. These airways are lined with mucus secreting columnar epithelium with cilia, designed to waft mucus towards the trachea. However, bronchioles are still too thick to allow gaseous exchange between air and blood.

Alveolar ducts and alveoli
The smallest bronchioles end in microscopic air sacs known as alveoli (from Latin *alveus* = hollow cavity). Alveoli form a large surface area of the lungs across which gases are exchanged. There are about 300 million alveoli in the two lungs. They have extremely thin walls. Nearly 90 per cent of surface is composed of squamous epithelium. The remaining 10 per cent of cells in this region is composed of septal cells that produce surfactant. Surfactant is a substance which reduces the surface tension of the water that moistens internal surfaces of the alveoli. It is of vital importance that these surfaces are moist, as oxygen will not diffuse into a dry surface. The alveoli are surrounded by a network of capillaries, through which the exchange of gases takes place between the air in the alveoli and blood in the capillaries.

Lungs
The lungs are two large spongy organs lying on the thorax on either side of the heart and great vessels. They are divided into lobes. The left lung has two lobes, each lobe consisting of five segments. These segments are referred to as bronchopulmonary segments. The right lung has three lobes broken down into ten segments. This division of the lungs into lobes plays an important role in the compartmentalisation of infections: for example, infection of lung tissue, pneumonia, is usually confined to a single lobe in the lung. The lungs are very light organs as the alveoli are filled with air.

Pulmonary circulation
Deoxygenated blood is transported to the lungs via the pulmonary arteries. Oxygenated blood returns to the heart via the pulmonary veins. These are the main vessels concerned with

carrying deoxygenated blood from the heart to the lungs and oxygenated blood from the lungs back to the heart.

Each segment of the lung is individually supplied with arterial blood via a pulmonary segmental artery.

An essential role of the lung is to maintain arterial blood–gas homeostasis. As part of this process, blood–gas composition is monitored continually by chemoreceptors. These chemorecptors are located in carotid and aortic arteries and in the brain (medulla region) and are sensory nerve endings which detect the gas composition of blood and feed this information back to the brain. This acts as an important homeostatic control.

Respiratory volumes and observation of respiration are addressed in Chapter 4.

The lymphatic system

The lymphatic system consists of capillaries, vessels, ducts and nodes that transport a fluid known as lymph. The lymphatic system is an extensive, branched tubular network that aligns itself with the blood circulation. Lymph is formed from the tissue fluid that surrounds all tissue cells. The lymphatic system performs three major functions:

1. transportation of lymphocytes
2. transportation of lipids
3. drainage of excess fluid from tissues.

Lymphatic capillaries
Unlike blood capillaries, the lymph capillaries are blind-ended; they are located in tissue spaces. Lymphatic capillaries are highly permeable and this allows them to absorb excess tissue fluid, proteins and micro-organisms. They are composed of endothelial cells, which are separated by pores that allow fluid to enter. Additionally, cells in the walls of lymphatic capillaries overlap to form valves, which promote the unidirectional (one-way) movement towards the neck region of the body, so lymph can be returned to the blood circulation. The flow of

lymph is very slow in comparison to blood; it is also regulated by lymphatic pumps and tissue pressure.

Lymph nodes consist of lymphatic channels held in place by connective tissue that forms a capsule. The nodes are packed with white blood cells (lymphocytes and macrophages) which can engulf foreign substances and micro-organisms. Macrophages act by phagocytosing (eating) bacteria. Lymph nodes are found throughout the body but are most common in the axilla (armpit) and groin.

The vessels carrying lymph away from the lymphatic nodes are referred to as efferent lymphatic vessels.

Other regions of lymphatic tissue
Lymphatic tissue is not only found in lymph nodes. It can be found in other locations throughout the body, including:

- spleen (located in the upper left portion of the abdomen)

- thymus gland (located in the chest)

- tonsil (located in the upper airway).

The immune system

When a foreign body (i.e. bacteria) is introduced into the body the immediate response is the production of a substance which will render it harmless. A foreign protein is called an antigen and substances produced in response to the antigen are called antibodies. The reaction that occurs in response to micro-organisms is called immunity. Immunity is a useful defence against infection.

There are two types of immunity in the human body:

1. cell-mediated immunity
2. antibody-mediated immunity.

Lymphocytes (T-cell and B-cell) are responsible for all cell- and antibody-mediated immunity. In response to an antigen, the lymphocytes produce T-cells, which attach themselves and ingest foreign bodies. These T-cells are able to recognise bacteria and viruses. B-cells produce specific protein molecules called antibodies, which also attach themselves to the antigen. By attaching themselves to the antigen, the lymphocytes render it inactive and the resulting immune complexes are later ingested by white blood cells. This complex process is of relevance to nurses as it enables humans to fight infection.

It is important that nurses understand the immunological homeostasis in the human body. The body's defences are continually operating to maintain intracellular integrity by combating harmful environmental agents (e.g. bacteria). It is estimated that up to one in ten patients entering hospital without an infection will suffer a hospital-acquired infection. It is a key nursing responsibility to prevent such occurrences.

The digestive system

Every day, the average adult consumes approximately 1kg of solid food and 1.2kg of fluid. In general, the form in which we eat food is unsuitable for immediate use by the body for growth, repair and the production of energy for the perfor-mance of physical work. During its passage though the gas-trointestinal tract, the food undergoes six processes:

1. ingestion
2. mastication
3. digestion
4. absorption
5. assimilation of useful components
6. elimination of non-usable residues.

The effect of the first three of these – ingestion, mastication and digestion – is to render the food into a state in which it can be absorbed. It is only at the fifth stage, assimilation, that food becomes of use to the body's cells. Substances which are not of use are eliminated at the final stage.

The adult gastrointestinal tract consists of a fibromuscular tube, approximately 4.5m long and of variable diameter, that extends from the mouth to the anus. The tract is in contact with the external environment at both ends, and as a result the potential problem exists of infective agents entering the body via this route. This problem is normally prevented by patches of protective lymphatic tissue throughout the tract.

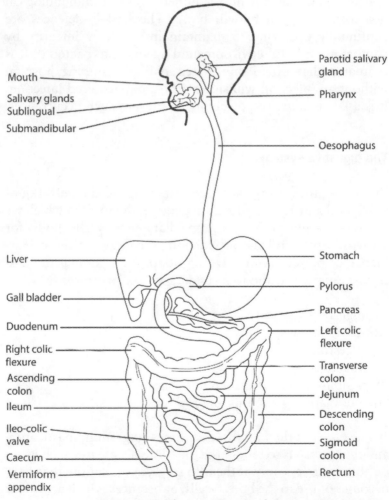

Figure 2.10 The gastrointestinal tract

The lips

The lips form a muscular entrance to the mouth. Lips are necessary for ingestion as they form a muscular passageway for food and fluids and help to grasp particles of food. Once food and fluids are in the mouth, the lips surround and usually close the entrance during chewing and swallowing. Clear speech in those with injured lips is extremely difficult. A further function of the lips is to convey information about the mood of the person – smiling, grimacing and kissing. The lips are covered by squamous, keratinised epithelial tissue which is very vascular and very sensitive.

The tongue

The tongue is formed of striated (voluntary) muscle which is anchored to the anterior floor of the mouth, behind the lower incisor teeth, by a fold of skin called the frenulum.

The tongue is very vascular and bleeds profusely when cut. It is also extremely sensitive, as it is supplied by a large number of nerve endings. If the tongue is injured in any way, then lisping and speech defects can result. Even a tiny lesion on the tongue can cause speech problems.

Apart from its function in speech, the tongue is necessary for swallowing ingested and masticated food. The tongue is very mobile and readily extensible and distensible. It also helps to mix food with saliva.

An important function of the tongue is that it allows us to taste and therefore derive enjoyment from food. On the superior surface of the tongue there are numerous papillae – variously called filiform, fungiform, circumvallate and foliate papillae according to their shape. These areas contain some 10,000 taste buds which allow us to differentiate between the four taste modalities – sweet, sour, salt and bitter.

The salivary glands

In terms of their contribution to digestion, these exocrine glands are non-essential; in practical terms, however, they are most important as their secretion aids speech, chewing, swallowing and general oral comfort. There are three main pairs of glands: the parotid glands, submaxillary and sub-lingual glands.

Saliva

Each day, adults produce approximately 1–1.5 litres of saliva. Saliva is formed mainly of water (99 per cent of total), and normally has a pH of 6.8–7.0.

Saliva has several functions:

- It cleans the mouth. There is a constant production of saliva with a backwards flow directed towards the oesophagus. Saliva contains lysozyme, which has an antiseptic action, and also immunoglobulin (IgA), which has a defensive function.

- It is necessary for chemicals in food to be in solution (i.e. mixed with saliva) for them to stimulate the taste receptors in the papillae on the tongue.

- Saliva is necessary for the formation of a food bolus.

Saliva contains a digestive enzyme, salivary amylase, which acts upon cooked starch (e.g. bread, pastry). It is produced in response to the following:

- *The thought, sight or smell of food.* This is a conditioned reflex. When a substance which is consciously recognised as food is anticipated by thought, sight or smell, impulses travel from the receptor to the cerebral cortex and thence to the medulla in the brainstem.

- *The presence of food in the mouth.* This produces mechanical stimulation of the salivary glands, and this response represents an unconditioned reflex (i.e. it is not learned).

Before digestion can occur, the ingested and masticated food (now in the form of a bolus) must be swallowed. This process is sometimes referred to as deglutition. The food is gathered into a bolus by the tongue, and before swallowing takes place the mouth is normally closed.

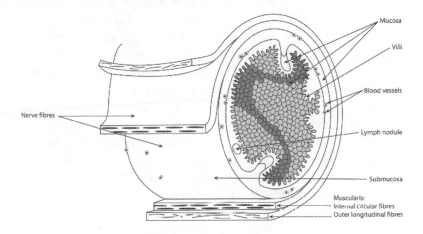

Figure 2.11 Layers of the gastrointestinal tract

Generalised structure of the gastrointestinal tract
The basic structure of the tract follows the same pattern from the mouth to the anus, with some functional adaptations throughout. The wall of the tube generally consists of four layers:

• The mucosa is the innermost layer.

• The submucosa lies distal to the mucosa, and consists of loose connective tissue which supports the blood vessels, lymphatics and nerves carried in this layer.

• The muscularis layer, as its name suggests, is formed of muscle fibres.

• The serosa is the outermost, protective layer, formed of connective tissue and squamous serous epithelium.

The oesophagus
Once food is in the oesophagus, or gullet, ring-like contractions propel it towards the stomach. This movement is called

peristalsis and is found throughout the gastrointestinal tract from the oesophagus to the colon. These movements occur progressively throughout the tube in a co-ordinated manner and give the appearance of smooth waves of contraction. The time taken for food to travel the 20–25cm of the oesophagus depends on the consistency of the food and the position of the body. Liquids take only 1–2 seconds to reach the stomach, but a more solid bolus takes longer, perhaps up to 2–3 minutes.

The lower section of the oesophagus is referred to as the gastro-oesophageal, or cardiac sphincter, and is normally in a state contraction until swallowing occurs, when the circular muscle fibres relax. This is a physiological rather than an anatomical sphincter; the circular muscles in the area act to prevent reflux of the gastric contents into the oesophagus.

Stomach

This is roughly J-shaped, although the size and shape vary between individuals and with its state of fullness. Its internal surface areas has visible folds called rugae, which together with the muscle layer allow distension. The epithelium of the body of the stomach (about 75 per cent of the total) is further folded, being composed of gastric pits containing microscopic gastric glands.

At rest, the volume of the 'empty' stomach in the adult is approximately 50ml. However, by receptive relaxation of the muscle in the stomach wall as food enters, it can accommodate up to 1.5 litres of food and fluids and under extreme circumstances can distend to hold nearly 4 litres.

Intrinsic factor is necessary for the absorption of Vitamin B_{12} in the small intestine. Vitamin B_{12} is required for healthy functioning of nerve fibres and for the formation of the red blood cells in the red bone marrow.

Ingested food is only partly broken down in the stomach, and the resulting molecules are still, in general, too large to cross the gastric wall. Hence only a small amount of absorption can occur in the stomach. It is possible to absorb the following:

- a small amount of water

- alcohol

- some drugs – in particular aspirin.

The stomach acts as a churn and converts ingested food to a thick minestrone soup-like consistency by mixing it with gastric secretions. The resulting semi-liquid substance is called chime.

Mixing is achieved by gastric peristalsis. Rhythmic waves of contraction of the three layers of smooth muscle in the stomach wall pass from cardia to pylorus about three times a minute, each wave lasting approximately half a minute. These waves of contraction allow the more liquid contents to leave the pylorus of the stomach quite rapidly and enter the duodenum.

Mucus consists of a gel, formed of the protein mucin, which adheres to the gastric mucosa. Mucus protects the stomach wall from being digested by the proteolytic enzyme pepsin, which is produced in the stomach (i.e. it prevents autodigestion). It helps to neutralise acid and further helps to lubricate the food in the stomach. In order to carry out these protective functions, the layer of mucus covering the rugae needs to be at least 1 mm thick.

Gastric juice consists of a mixture of secretions from two types of cells:

- Parietal or oxyntic cells – these secrete hydrochloric acid (HCI) and also the intrinsic factor referred to earlier.

- Chief or zymogen cells – these secrete enzymes.

Some 2–3 litres of juice with a pH of 1.5–3.0 are secreted each day in the adult. The functions of gastric acid are as follows:

- It inactivates salivary amylase.

- It is bacteriostatic and therefore protective.

- It denatures proteins; that is, it alters their molecular structure.

- It converts pepsinogen into pepsin.

The chief (or zymogen) cells produce a scanty secretion rich in pepsinogen, an enzyme precursor. While gastric pH is below 5.5, this pepsinogen is converted into pepsin by hydrochloric acid. Once this conversion has occurred, the pepsin so formed can itself convert pepsinogen into more pepsin. Pepsin is a proteolytic enzyme; that is, it acts on proteins and starts their digestion.

Control of gastric-juice secretion is under both neural and hormonal controls. It is usual to describe two phases in the neural control of gastric juice secretion, although these two phases are not distinct.

In the cephalic, secretion is brought about in response to the sight, thought or smell of food. This is a conditioned (i.e. learned) reflex, and is mediated by the vagus nerve. Additionally, the presence of food in the mouth leads to gastric secretion. The gastric phase is not mediated by the vagus nerve. The presence of food in the stomach produces mechanical stimuli which result in gastric-juice secretion. Stretch receptors in the stomach wall respond to distension of the stomach wall, and chemoreceptors to protein molecules within the stomach. Hormonal influences also contribute to the gastric phase of gastric-juice secretion.

A small amount of *gastrin* is produced by the duodenal mucosa. This production is sometimes referred to as the intestinal phase of the control of gastric-juice secretion.

Gastrin is secreted in response to the presence in the stomach of certain foodstuffs referred to as secretagogues, examples of which are meat, alcohol, tea, coffee and colas, and also in response to the acetylcholine release as a result of vagal stimulation. Once produced, gastrin enters the gastric capillaries and then the systemic circulation. When it reaches the stomach via the bloodstream it:

- stimulates the parietal cells to produce gastric acid by liberating histamine

- has a minor role in stimulating the chief cells to produce pepsinogen

- stimulates the growth of the gastric and intestinal mucosa

- brings about enhanced contraction of the cardiac sphincter, and hence prevents reflux during gastric activity

- stimulates the secretion of insulin and glucagon when it reaches the pancreas via the systemic circulation.

The time that foods remain in the stomach depends upon their consistency and composition. Carbohydrate foodstuffs, together with liquids, leave fastest; then protein-based foods; and finally fatty foods are the slowest to leave the stomach.

The small intestine
The small intestine is approximately 3.0–3.5m long in the adult and consists of three sections:

- The C-shaped duodenum, which is 20–25cm long.

- The jejunum (meaning empty) forms approximately 40 per cent of the remainder of the small intestine.

- The ileum (meaning twisted) is a slightly longer tube making up the final 60 per cent.

The function of the small intestine is to complete the digestion of ingested food and to absorb practically all the nutrients and most of the water from the chyme, which enters this area from the gastrointestinal tract. The duodenum receives the secretions of the pancreatic and common bile duct at a point called the sphincter of Oddi, which lies about 10cm below the pylorus. The secretions produced by both the pancreas and the liver and delivered to the duodenum are alkaline, having a pH in the range 7.8–8.4. There is therefore a sharp change in the pH of the intestinal contents (from the gastric pH of 1.5–3.0) after the addition of bile and pancreatic juice to the duodenal pH of approximately 7.0. The digestive enzymes in the small intestine are, like all enzymes, pH specific (that is, there is a critical pH for their optimal activity) and act best at a pH of 6.5–7.0.

The pancreas has a major role in digestion. Its exocrine digestive function is served by acinar cells, which structurally resemble cells of the salivary glands. These cells form and store zymogen granules, which consist of protein-based digestive enzymes. These enzymes are discharged in response to stimulation, mainly hormonal, and are secreted into the pancreatic duct. This duct joins with the common bile duct to form a slightly dilated area called the ampulla of Vater, which then empties into the duodenum via the sphincter of Oddi.

Between 1.5 and 2 litres of pancreatic juice are secreted daily with a pH of 8.0–8.4. Three digestive enzymes are produced by the acinar cells of the pancreas trypsinogen, pancreatic amylase and lipase. For the reason described earlier in relation to pepsin – namely, to prevent autodigestion – they are secreted in the inactive form.

Trypsinogen is converted into the active form trypsin by the enzyme enterokinase (also called enteropeptidase) secreted by the duodenal mucosa. Trypsin acts on proteins and polypeptides, breaking bonds between the amino acids and thus forming short sections of amino acid units). Trypsin, once formed, has three further actions:

1. It activates trypsinogen to form more trypsin.
2. It activates chymotrypsinogen to form chymotrypsin, which has the same proteolytic functions as trypsin.
3. In addition, trypsin activates procarboxypeptidase to form active carboxypeptidase.

Pancreatic juice also contains pancreatic amylase and lipase, which act on carbohydrates and fats respectively.

Intestinal juice is secreted by the jejunum and ileum. The enzymes present in intestinal juice are responsible for the completion of digestion. Up to 3 litres of this secretion, with a pH of 7.8–8.0, are normally produced each day by the small intestine in response to local mechanical stimuli and to the chemical stimuli of partially digested food products on the intestinal mucosa. In addition, secretion of intestinal juice is stimulated by emotional disturbances.

The surface area of the small intestine is increased by visible folding of the mucosa into valvulae conniventes and by the presence of finger-like processes, each about 0.5mm long, called *villi*. These features serve to increase the surface area to 600 times that of a non-folded tube of the same length. The total surface area is further increased by the presence of microvilli on the villous surfaces. The mucosa of the small intestine is invaginated between adjacent villi to form pits, called the crypts of Lieberkühn, where the mucus-secreting glands are located.

There are 20–40 villi/mm^2 of the intestinal mucosa. Each villus consists of a finger-like process, the surface of which is covered by simple columnar epithelium continuous with that of the crypts. Within each villus there is a central lacteal which contains lymph and which empties into the local lymphatic circulation; each also has a capillary blood supply which links with both the hepatic and portal veins. The surface of the villus is usually covered with a layer of mucus, which prevents autodigestion by proteolytic enzymes.

Villi contain two main cell types: the goblet cells, secreting mucus and situated mainly in the crypts, and the enterocytes, which are involved in both digestion and absorption. Enterocytes are tall columnar cells, their nuclei lying towards their bases. Their surfaces are each covered with up to 3000 microvilli, which increase the villous surface area. These microvilli give what is known as a brush border to the villus. Enterocytes have many mitochondria to provide for the high-energy demands of enzyme secretion and absorption.

Enzymes present in the enterocyte membrane:

- Aminopeptidases acts on long chain proteins (peptides).

- Dipeptidases act on dipeptides (i.e. units of two joined amino acids) and break them into single amino acids.

- Maltase acts on maltose to convert it into glucose.

- Lactase acts on lactose to convert it into glucose and galactose.

- Sucrase acts on sucrose to convert it into glucose and fructose.

In summary, digestion is now complete and ingested food has been rendered into a form in which it can be absorbed.

- Proteins have been broken down into amino acids.

- Fats have been broken down into fatty acids and glycerol.

- Carbohydrates have been broken down into monosaccharides – glucose, fructose and galactose.

Absorption
Each day, approximately 8–9 litres of water and 1kg of nutrients pass across the wall of the gut from its lumen into its blood supply. This process requires energy, which is derived from the breakdown of glucose and fatty acids.

Transport of nutrients across the cell membranes of the gastrointestinal epithelial cells can be either active or passive.

- *Active transport.* This requires the expenditure of energy.

- *Passive transport.* This requires no energy consumption. Water, lipids, drugs and some electrolytes and vitamins are examples of substances transported passively from the gut into the blood.

Absorption of nutrients and minerals including proteins, carbohydrates and fats occurs in this region.

The large intestine
In an adult, the large intestine is approximately 1.5m long and consists of the caecum, appendix, colon and rectum
The large intestine has five functions:

1. storage of food residues prior to their elimination
2. absorption of most of the remaining water, electrolytes and some vitamins
3. synthesis of Vitamin K and some B vitamins by colonic bacteria
4. secretion of mucus, which acts as a lubricant for the elimination of faeces
5. elimination of food residues as faeces.

Each day, about one litre of chyme enters the large intestine via the ileocaecal valve. The ileocaecal valve opens in response to peristaltic waves which bring chyme into contact with it. In addition, when food enters the stomach, a reflex is set up via the vagus nerve which stimulates peristalsis in the colon. This causes the caecum to relax and the ileocaecal valve to open. This reflex is called the gastrocolic reflex. The consequent colonic peristalsis causes the rectum to fill with faeces, and this results in the urge to defaecate.

The large intestine has no villi, and hence has a much smaller internal surface area – approximately one-third that of the small intestine.

The appendix is a worm-like blind-ending sac projecting from the end of the caecum, and about the size of an adult's little finger. It is made up mainly of lymphoid tissue and can enlarge in infection or inflammation (appendicitis).

The colon is a dilated area of the large intestine and is anatomically divided into several regions:

• ascending colon

- transverse colon

- descending colon

- sigmoid colon.

The colon differs from the generalised structure of the gastrointestinal tract described earlier in that the longitudinal muscle bands in the muscularis layer are incomplete.

The main function of the colon is to store unabsorbed food residues. The colon thus acts as a reservoir; 70 per cent of the residue of food is excreted within 72 hours of ingestion, and the remaining 30 per cent can stay within the colon for a week or longer.

Segmentation allows mixing of the colonic contents and facilitates colonic absorption. Peristalsis, described earlier, also occurs in the colon, propelling faeces towards the rectum.

The rectum is a muscular tube about 12–15cm long, capable of great distension. It is usually empty until just before defaecation. The rectum opens to the exterior via the anal canal, which has both internal and external anal sphincters. The internal anal sphincter is composed of smooth muscle fibres and is not under voluntary control. The external anal sphincter is composed of striated muscle fibres and is under the control of the will from about the age of 18 months. Defaecation is thus a reflex response to faeces entering the rectum. Approximately 100–150g of faeces are usually eliminated every day, consisting of 30–50g of solids and 70–100g of water.

The urinary system

The urinary system is composed of the organs and structures which produce, transport and store urine. It consists of:

- the kidneys

- the ureters

- the bladder

- the urethra.

The kidneys form the urine, which is then stored in the urinary bladder, and is eliminated from the body in a controlled process. There are two kidneys in the human body situated high in the abdominal cavity, one on each side of the vertebral column. The right kidney lies a little lower than the left as a consequence of the position of the liver. Each weighs about 150g and is described as a red, bean-shaped organ.

Surrounding the outer surface of each kidney is a layer of connective tissue, the renal capsule. The kidney has two distinct regions, a darker outer layer of the kidney called the cortex and the paler inner portion called the renal medulla. The cortex is composed of extremely vascular tissue that supports the production of urine, by a process called filtration. The renal medulla is composed of structures called renal pyramids.

Within each kidney there are approximately one million minute twisted tubules called nephrons. Nephrons are the functional unit of the kidney and do the bulk of the work. Each nephron consists of a renal tubule and an associated vascular system. The first part of the renal tubule is called the Bowman's (glomerular) capsule; this is located in the cortex of the kidney. Within the cup of each capsule comes a fine branch of the renal artery, forming a ball of capillaries called the glomerulus. Glomerular capillaries are located inside the glomerular capsule. The glomerulus and the glomerular capsule are referred to as a renal corpuscle.

The arteriole supplying blood to the glomerulus is known as the afferent, and the arteriole which carries the blood away is known as the efferent vessel. The efferent vessel is slightly smaller than the afferent vessel.

The next section of the renal tubule is termed the proximal convoluted (= coiled) tubule which leads into the loop of

Henle, which dips down into the medulla and then passes back into the cortex. This rises again, back towards the cortex, where it forms into the distal convoluted tubule before connecting to a collecting duct.

Formation of urine

The main function of the kidneys is to secrete and excrete urine. To maintain renal homeostasis, urine formation must regulate the removal of harmful waste products and conserve water and electrolytes in the body. Urine is produced by three processes:

1. filtration
2. reabsorption
3. secretion.

Endothelial cells of the glomerular capillaries contain small pores, podocytes and pedicels, which are too small to allow blood to pass through. This acts as a filter and fluid and smaller components may pass out of the capillaries via these pores. This fluid is known as glomerular filtrate and is composed of glucose, amino acids, fatty acids and urea. As highlighted in Chapter 4, blood cells and protein molecules are only filtered if the kidney is diseased. Each kidney receives 600 mls of blood per minute producing 125ml of glomerular filtrate. As the average amount of urine passed each day is about 1.5 litres, a degree of reabsorption of filtration is required.

Reabsorption

As glomerular filtrate passes through the nephron 99 per cent is reabsorbed back into the blood. Selective reabsorption occurs because the cells which line the convoluted tubules have the ability to absorb water, glucose, salt and electrolytes that the body requires. Reabsorption of water in the distal convoluted tubule is controlled by secretion of anti-diuretic hormone (ADH) from the posterior lobe of the pituitary gland. A decrease in secretion of ADH results in less water being reabsorbed, therefore more water is excreted as urine. Aldos-terone, a hormone produced in the adrenal cortex, is one of the main controls of reabsorption of salts. Nervous and hormonal (adrenalin and noradrenalin) controls regulate blood pressure in the glomerular capillaries to ensure filtration takes place.

Composition of urine

Normal urine is about 95 per cent water and 5 per cent dissolved solutes. It is an amber-coloured fluid in colour according to its concentration. The colour of urine comes from the breakdown of bile. It should always be transparent; if it is cloudy, this may indicate the presence of bacteria.

Urine consists of water, salts and protein waste products (urea and creatinine). The average composition is:

Water	96%
Urea	2%
Salts	2%

The percentage of urea in the blood is 0.04 per cent as opposed to 2 per cent in urine. This clearly demonstrates the effect the kidney has on concentration. The salt composition of urine consists chiefly of sodium, potassium, calcium, chlorides, phosphates and sulphates. Normal urine may also include ketones, a breakdown product of fat metabolism; this is parti-cularly noted if an individual has not eaten for a period of time.

A good example of homeostatic control within the urinary system relates to the control of water balance. If we do not drink enough fluid, receptors in the brain (osmoreceptors and thirst receptors) are stimulated and we are induced to drink fluids, which is a behavioural response mediated through the nervous system.

At the same time an anti-diuretic hormone is released from the brain and it acts to reduce the production of urine and thereby reduces the volume of water lost from the body. Once again this illustrates that the homeostatic processes are con-stantly working within all the systems of the body to maintain a stable environment.

Integumentary system

The skin, hair, nails and glands make up the integumentary system. Its main functions include protection of the body, regulation of body temperature, elimination of waste, sensation and production of Vitamin D. In this section the structure and the function of skin will be examined.

The structure of the skin
The skin is the largest organ in the body; it consists of two layers, the outer epidermis and the inner dermis. Skin surface area varies from one individual to the next, but in most adults it covers about 1.5 to 2 square metres. The skin protects us from the environment and plays a major role in temperature regulation. In its protective role, it prevents the body from dehydration, resists the invasion of micro-organisms and provides protection from the harmful effects of ultraviolet rays in sunlight.

The *epidermis* forms the outer layer of the body and is comprised of stratified squamous epithelium, which can be subdivided into five distinct layers:

1. basal layer (= stratum basale)
2. layer of 'prickly' cells (= stratum spinosum)
3. layer of 'granular' cells (= stratum granulosum)
4. layer of 'cornified' cells (= stratum corneum)
5. layer of 'clear' cells (= stratum lucidium).

Only areas of skin exposed to considerable wear and tear, such as the soles of the feet, have the fifth layer between the granular and cornified layers, stratum lucidium.

The cells of the outer layer of the epidermis are said to be keratinised because they contain the waterproof protein keratin, which gives the epidermis its ability to protect the underlying dermis.

There are no blood vessels with the epidermis itself. The demands of the cells in the epidermis are met by blood vessels within the dermis. The turnover of cells from the deeper layers of the epidermis to the surface means that the upper layer of skin is constantly being regenerated. The approximate time for turnover of the epidermis is typically about eight weeks.

The *dermis* is a connective tissue that contains several types of structures, including collagen fibres, elastin fibres, nerve endings, blood and lymphatic vessels. The spaces between fibres contain many of the appendages associated with the skin.

The skin carries four main appendages:

1. sweat glands
2. hairs
3. nails
4. sebaceous glands.

Functions of the skin
The main functions of the skin are as follows:

● to regulate body temperature

● to secrete waste products

● to act as the organ of touch and other senses

● to protect us from bacteria

● to secrete sebum

● to protect the body from the harmful effects of sunlight

● to produce Vitamin D.

Body temperature is regulated between heat gained and heat lost. It is essential that body temperature is finely controlled, as many of the biochemicals found in human beings only work within narrow ranges of temperature. Therefore if the body becomes too hot or cold, homeostasis will be disrupted. Humans are classified as warm-blooded animals and their temperature must be maintained around 37°C; any deviation affects the normal functioning of the nervous system and enzymes.

The core temperature in the body relates to the temperature in the main organs. Core temperature remains constant over long periods of time, although it does vary slightly through a 24-hour period. It is normally about 0.5°C below normal first thing in the morning and can rise as much as 1.0°C higher later in the day. Peripheral temperature relates to the body temperature on the surface of the skin or in the hands and feet. This may be lower than the core temperature, especially in colder climes.

The main temperature regulating region is the hypothalamus, situated within the brain.

The hypothalamus acts as via a negative feedback pathway; if the body temperature rises, mechanisms come into action so that heat is lost from the body. There are several mechanisms of heat loss, including:

- radiation, conduction and convection of heat from the skin

- evaporation

- respiration

- excretion of urine and faeces.

The rate of heat generation is determined mainly through metabolic activity.

The liver, as a large metabolically active organ, produces a great deal of heat. The levels of thyroid hormone in the body are also a major determinant of metabolic rate.

Additional heat is produced by:

- exercise

- activity

- shivering

- infection

- trauma (e.g. burns)

- emotion.

Heat production is lowest during sleep and highest during physical activity.

Normal body temperature varies a little from individual to individual. However, a temperature of 37°C is considered normal. A temperature in excess of 37.5°C is usually indicative of some form of infection or tissue damage. During exercise body temperature may rise to above of 38°C. However, this rise triggers cooling responses, such as sweating.

If the environment is very cold then body temperature may start to drop. Older people are particularly prone to reduced body temperatures. If the body temperature drops below 35°C, this may be described as hypothermia.

Hypothermia normally arises from prolonged exposure to cold environments, but a tendency towards hypothermia is noted in people with lowered metabolic activity (e.g. deficient in thyroid hormone). The effects of hypothermia on metabolic rate include a reduced heart rate, lethargy and slower reflexes. Neurological and cardiac functions decline with progressive hypothermia, which can lead to death. Nursing care of the hypothermic patient is discussed in Chapter 4.

FURTHER READING

The following textbooks have been consulted in the preparation of this chapter:

Campbell, J. (2003) *Campbell's Physiology Notes for Nurses*, London: Whurr.
Clancy, J. and McVicar, A. J. (2002) *Physiology and Anatomy: A Homeostatic Approach*, 2nd edn, London: Arnold. See esp. chs 8, 10–15.

Hinchliff, S., Montague, S. and Watson, R. (1996) *Physiology for Nursing Practice*, 2nd edn, London: Bailliere Tindall. See esp. chs 2, 4–9.

Marieb, E. N. (2001) *Human Anatomy and Physiology*, 5th edn, San Francisco: Longman.

Tortura, G. J. and Grabowski, S. R. (2003) *Principles of Anatomy Physiology*, 10th edn, New York: Wiley.

Watson, R. (2000) *Anatomy and Physiology for Nurses*, 11th edn, London: Bailliere Tindall. See esp. chs 5, 15–17, 18–21, 24.

Watson, R. (1999) *Essential Science for Nursing Students: An Introductory Text*, London: Bailliere Tindall.

3 SOCIAL SCIENCES IN NURSING

WHAT IS PSYCHOLOGY?

In everyday conversation the term psychology is widely used and often confused with psychiatry, which is the study of mental disorders. The word 'psychology' comes from two words: psyche and logos. *Psyche* originates from the Greek language and can be loosely translated as 'mind'. *Logos* means study or knowledge. Therefore, in the most basic of terms, psychology can be defined as the study of the mind. However, in practice, psychology also relates to what is observable and measurable in a person's behaviour, including the biological processes in the body. A more comprehensive definition of psychology is therefore: the scientific study of the mind and the behaviour of humans and animals.

Unlike the biological sciences, psychology does not have one unifying theory or approach. There are several psychological perspectives or theories, including:

- humanistic

- psychodynamic

- behavioural

- cognitive

- bio-psychological.

In psychology these theories are used to make predictions or to understand how people think and behave. These theories are explored later in this chapter.

In addition to different theories or perspectives within psychology student nurses will notice that the subject of psychology within the university departments is often divided into separate areas of study. These may include:

• developmental psychology

• social psychology

• comparative psychology

• individual differences

• cognitive psychology

• health psychology.

Therefore psychology is a vast subject area and in this chapter it will only be possible to touch on the topic areas that are of most relevance to nurse education. One area of importance to nurses, is that of health psychology, which has only evolved in recent years. Health psychology is a discipline which links the principles of psychology to health-care practice.

Nursing has become increasingly based upon the knowledge of scientific principles. Social sciences, such as psychology and sociology, are important components of nurse education in the twenty-first century. Many university-based nursing courses include elements of psychology and sociology with their curriculum. The relevance of psychology may not be imme-diately apparent to the potential nursing student. It is the study of experience which makes psychology relevant and of interest to nurses. Nurses should be aware that to function as a person involves psychological and social aspects, as well as fully functioning body systems, as described in Chapter 2. This section highlights the value of a psychological understanding in nursing care in relation to interpersonal care and covers the following areas:

- psychology in health care

- understanding ourselves/self

- perspectives/theories of psychology

- stress

- pain.

Humanistic psychology in particular focuses on the uniqueness of the experiencing self and views this as more important than merely observing behaviour and making generalisations. An awareness of basic psychology allows nurses to make more sense of the lives of their patients whom they care for and extend the range of ways that they can help them. For example, a newly diagnosed patient with cancer may have psychological difficulties, such as fear of the unknown, or occupational, financial and marital difficulties, which may lead to feelings of anxiety and depression to compound their physical symptoms.

Due to the brevity of this section readers are encouraged to refer to basic introductory psychology textbooks for additional information where appropriate.

PSYCHOLOGY IN HEALTH CARE

Nurses spend a great deal of their time working with people from all walks of life:

- patients

- relatives

- other nurses

- doctors

- other hospital staff

- students.

Working in a health-care setting, whether in a hospital or in the community, involves understanding not only how individuals function but how they interact with each other. Psychology is of interest to nurses because its subject matter is that of human behaviour. As identified above, nurses interact with a variety of people every moment of their working day and in many instances these people may behave in a manner which is difficult to understand or undesirable. In order for nurses to deal effectively with these situations nurses must first understand their own behaviour and attitudes.

There are several reasons why nurses need to have an understanding of psychological theories. First, to understand fully the needs of potentially vulnerable groups in society, such as, the sick, elderly, children, those with learning difficulties, socially and economically disadvantaged, to name but a few of these groups. Second, the nurse should be aware of the impact of long-term chronic illness. Patients with chronic illnesses such as cardiovascular diseases, cancer and respiratory disorders are people who are likely to require long-term care and treatment which may influence their ability to function as normal. The impact that a chronic disease has upon an individual's work, social activities and relationships may have a detrimental effect upon his or her quality of life. It is important for the nurse to be fully aware of these psychosocial consequences of illness. Third, it is important for nurses to recognise the link between lifestyle and health. Whether through excessive smoking, alcohol consumption, diet or sexual behaviour, an individual's lifestyle or behaviour can influence their health status.

UNDERSTANDING OURSELVES

Before we attempt to understand the behaviour and thought processes of others, it is of relevance to examine our understanding of ourselves. Nurses need to understand what it is to be a professional carer and to understand their own motivation for wishing to care and to be able to disentangle their own thoughts and emotions from those of the individuals they care for. Self-concept is the knowledge that a person has about himself/herself. It makes up the information that we acquire through interactions with others and consists of an organised set of beliefs and feelings that are self-referent. The self-concept influences how we process information about the external social world in relation to ourselves. Carl Rogers, a humanistic psychologist, particularly emphasised the role of self-concept, which he believed comprises three parts:

- self-image

- ideal self

- self-esteem.

Self-image relates to how we perceive ourselves. Ideal self relates to how we would like to perceive ourselves. Self-esteem reflects a critical evaluative judgement of self-worth. It is based on a combination of how we perceive others see us, together with our own appraisal of these judgements. Self-esteem has a major role to play in the psychological well-being of people and as such it is important for nurses to be aware of this concept.

Nurses need to access their own thoughts, feelings and motivation for behaviour so as to give them an awareness of how they may respond to the thoughts, feelings, beliefs and behaviours of others. It would be difficult for nurses to demonstrate a positive regard and sense of value towards their patients without first being aware of the self. Self-awareness can be defined as bringing into consciousness various aspects of our understanding of ourselves and allows for the analysis of motives for behaviour.

To understand further the motivation for behaviour, Abraham Maslow, a humanistic psychologist, devised the 'hierarchy of needs'. This provides a framework for the needs of life and predicts that there is an order in which needs have to be satisfied to enable individuals to achieve self-actualisation. Self-actualisation is an innate human motivation whereby each of us has to reach our full potential by using and developing our talents and abilities. The lower levels of Maslow's scale identify the requirements related to physical safety, such as food and shelter, and progresses through to love and self-esteem, reaching to the pinnacle of self-actualisation. The hierarchy forms part of a theory which proposes that lower-level needs must be met before higher-level needs can be fulfilled.

In summary, when working with vulnerable groups in our society, nurses who have an insight into their own thoughts, feelings and behaviours are more likely to understand what motivates the attitudes and behaviours of others. An understanding of the self is essential to facilitate this process of analysis. Through an understanding of their own motivations for behaviour, their own responses to stress and the origins of attitudes and prejudices, nurses will be better positioned to understand individuals in their care.

PERSPECTIVES OF PSYCHOLOGY

The following section introduces some of the main theoretical perspectives in psychology. Different perspectives of psychology represent different spheres of interest and different ways of interpreting events. Although the surface is merely scratched on these perspectives within this text, it is important for nurses to be informed on the variety of psychological theories to aid human understanding.

Psychodynamic/psychoanalytic

The term 'psychodynamic' relates to an active mind. Sigmund Freud (1856–1939) coined the term psychoanalysis to describe his theories and techniques for treating the mental problems of his patients. He viewed the mind in three states, that is, conscious, pre-conscious and unconscious:

- Conscious: awareness we have when we are awake

- Pre-conscious: boundary between conscious and unconscious

- Unconscious: containing our secret wishes and fears; these thoughts are completely hidden to us.

According to Freud, the mind has three processes, each with its own motives and developmental progress. These three mental processes – the id, the ego and the superego – interact to help us survive.

The id is the most basic part of the personality. It is inborn and develops alone for the first couple of years of life. The id is involved in the satisfaction of the most basic of instincts and operates by the 'pleasure principle'. For example, babies usually seek pleasure (e.g. food, drink, comfort and warmth) and avoid the unpleasurable (e.g. hunger, being wet and cold). The id is selfish and typically wants immediate gratification.

The ego develops from around the age of two years and operates by the 'reality principle', the part of the personality which balances the fulfilment of basic instincts with what is socially acceptable. The id cannot be allowed to have its own way, so the ego often has to battle with it. Freud claimed that it was a mistake for the ego always to inhibit the id and believed that people should sometimes 'let go' and enjoy themselves. If this does not occur, he maintained that our id could become very frustrated and possibly achieve its own way at the wrong place or time.

The superego acts as a social conscience in our mind. It

starts to develop about the age of three under the influence of parental figures. It develops throughout childhood, becoming fully mature after puberty. The 'super' of this process means 'above' and relates to the superego looking down or monitoring the id and the ego. The superego is our 'moral watchdog', which prevents us from doing wrong, especially with regard to being anti-social. Whereas the id and ego are selfish, the superego has consideration for others.

According to Freud, there are five stages of psychosexual development that we pass through:

1. oral phase 0–2 years
2. anal phase 2–3 years
3. phallic phase 3–6 years
4. latent phase 6–11 years
5. genital phase 11+ years.

During the oral phase the mouth is the prime source of pleasure, for survival. The baby instinctively sucks, from which it obtains pleasure. Through oral satisfaction, the baby develops trust and an optimistic personality. If there is a lack of oral stimulation (i.e. if we are weaned too early) there is a risk of being stuck at this stage, described as 'oral fixation'. Freud believed that the personality of a baby in oral fixation may become pessimistic or aggressive.

The locus of attention shifts to the anus during the second and third years of life. The child becomes aware of its bowels and how to control them. The focus here is on toilet training and the child can choose to give or withhold faeces in order to provide pleasure. By deciding itself, the child takes an important step of independence. However, overly strict parents who force the child to go to the toilet and demand cleanliness may lead to personality problems, depending on how the child reacts. Freud believed difficulties during this phase could lead to anal fixation. The child who is forced to go to the toilet may become reluctant to give anything away and develop an anally retentive personality. Similarly, over concern about going regularly to the toilet during this phase may cause an individual to become either an obsessive time-keeper or an extremely poor time-keeper.

During the phallic phase the child becomes aware of their genitals and sexual differences. Consequently, development is different for boys and girls. Freud proposed that during this phase of development, boys fantasise about their mothers and girls fantasise about their fathers. In boys this reaction is known as the Oedipus complex. These three phases of early-years development are thought to be particularly important to personality development.

Sexual development takes place in two phases: a pre-genital phase and a genital phase which usually begins at puberty. These phases of sexual development are distinguished by whether or not the genital zones have assumed a dominating role. Between these two phases there is a lull or period of latency. Latency may be total or partial, and during this period sexual inhibitions can develop.

Repression is not a conscious process but a mechanism by which the ego protects itself from threatening events. Unwanted thoughts or ideas are pushed into the unconscious mind and stored there. This is a defence mechanism by which unpleasant, guilty, horrible and frightening thoughts are avoided. However, too much repression can lead to mental problems, as it can be exhausting. Psychoanalytic psychologists argue that it is better for unpleasant thoughts to rise into the conscious mind so that they can be dealt with. Psychoanalytic theory is mainly used by psychologists to treat patients who have emotional problems, such as anxiety and depression. This therapy is based upon talking about past memories and experiences, particularly those which occurred in childhood and may have been repressed.

Other defence mechanisms described by Freud include:

• Regression – going back to an earlier stage to find comfort (e.g. thumb-sucking).

• Displacement – diverting energy (libido) on to another activity.

- Sublimation – getting rid of stress or anxiety positively (e.g. sport).

Freud's theories and methods have been modified and adapted by post-Freudian psychologists including Carl Jung and Erik Erikson. There remains to this day a degree of controversy surrounding psychoanalytic theory. It is criticised as being unscientific and untestable. The use of psychoanalytic theory in nursing is mostly seen in psychiatry.

Behavioural approaches

When patients are unconscious, or too ill to speak, their behaviour may be the only way that nurses can tell if they are in discomfort or pain. A behavioural approach involves the investigation of the way that people learn, based upon observations of how they respond in different circumstances to different types of consequence. Learning can be defined as a relatively permanent change in behaviour due to experience. Perhaps the most famous behavioural experiment was conducted by the Russian physiologist Ivan Pavlov. He demonstrated the principle of classic conditioning in his studies with dogs. Pavlov knew that dogs, like humans, salivate in the presence of food. This salivation is a natural reflex response. As such, food can be seen as an unconditioned stimulus and salivation is an unconditioned response. Pavlov demonstrated that if a bell was rung immediately prior to giving a dog food, the dog would eventually salivate as soon as the bell was rung, before it saw the food. Salivation to a bell is not a natural, but a conditioned reflex. Therefore the bell is a conditioned stimulus and salivation to the bell is a conditioned response. Pavlov termed this classical conditioning, or reflex learning, and it takes place at a subconscious level. This classic-conditioning theory enables health professionals to understand the development of many fears and phobias. For example, the arachnophobic views the spider (stimulus) as anxiety-provoking and leads to panic in the presence of a spider (response).

The founding father of behaviourism, John Watson, viewed emotions as simple environmental stimuli with measurable responses. For example, the nurse may detect that a patient is anxious if that individual has an increased pulse rate or is sweating.

The other main behaviourist theory is that of operant conditioning devised by Burrhus Skinner. He mainly studied voluntary behaviour in humans and developed a theory on the role of reinforcement (positive consequences) and punishment (aversive consequences) of behaviour. Not all psychologists believed that human behaviour could be explained by stimulus, response, reinforcement and punishment. It is important to also examine the cognitive (mental) processes.

Cognitive

An alternative approach to understanding people's behaviour is to consider their thought processes. A cognitive approach basically relates to thinking and how we perceive events, memory, language, intelligence and problem-solving. Cognitive therapy was initially developed in the early 1960s by Dr Aaron Beck of the University of Pennsylvania in the United States. Cognitive approaches takes an information-processing approach to individuals based on the premise that the way people interpret their experiences determines the way they feel and act.

Humanistic psychology

The focus of humanistic psychology is on the here and now, on the concept of self. Humanistic psychology developed from phenomenology, the study of immediate experience as it occurs, and it is the precursor of a field of psychological study known as Gestalt. The main bases of humanistic psychology are:

1. a focus on the individual, especially free will and personal choice
2. emphasis on the conscious experience
3. the wholeness of human nature.

Humanistic psychologists criticise behaviourist psychologists for reducing humans to programmable machines. They also disagree with Freud's emphasis on the negative aspects of mental illness, whilst humanists concentrate more on the positive attributes of mental health, such as happiness, contentment, caring and sharing. Carl Rogers is the psychologist most commonly associated with humanistic psychology and he developed a concept of self-actualisation influenced by Maslow. Rogers worked with people with emotional problems and rejected both behaviourist and psychoanalytic perspectives. He believed that self-actualisation is an innate tendency, which drives everyone to achieve his or her full potential. He noted that many of the individuals who came to him with psychological concerns exhibited a natural tendency towards personal growth and maturity to deal with their own problems. Rogers developed person-centred therapy in the belief that if individuals are given the correct environment, opportunity and freedom, they can identify their own solutions to their problems. Many of these psychological problems have their origin in childhood. He identified three particular qualities as playing an important part in this therapeutic relationship. These are known as the core conditions:

1. Empathetic understanding – the ability to imagine what someone is feeling.
2. Genuineness or congruence – relates to being open or honest in a relationship.
3. Unconditional positive regard – accepting clients as fellow humans entitled to care and respect.

The requirement for these three qualities was first identified in the context of a counselling relationship. He believed these

three qualities were necessary and sufficient to enable con-
structive personality change. This psychological perspective
has had a considerable influence upon the nursing profession
as it aims to give power back to the clients, or patients,
empowering them to make their own decisions and promote
psychological growth. Humanistic psychology is relevant to
nursing as it places focus on the uniqueness of the experiencing
self and views this as important as observing behaviours or
making generalisations.

An important way in which we develop our own sense of
ourselves occurs by comparing ourselves with other people
and building up images of what we would like to be. George
Kelly was the founder of personal construct theory within the
humanistic tradition. Humanistic psychological approaches
which facilitate listening to individuals and providing them
with an opportunity to disclose worries and fears has become
very popular within health care and in particular within
nursing. Counselling and listening skills are commonly incorporated within nursing courses.

STRESS

Understanding the concept of stress is important for nurses as
it will often reveal how people perceive and respond to
changes in their health status. In nursing it is of value to look
at the causes of stress as stimuli, or stressors, and to view stress
itself as the reaction or response to the stimuli. As no two
patients will necessarily respond in the same way to identical
stimuli, nurses can only really determine whether an event or
experience is perceived as stressful by the patient by observing
the reaction of that particular individual. Equally individual is
the manner in which stress is dealt with; this is termed
'coping'.

The term 'stress' has many connotations and definitions
based on a variety of perspectives of the human condition. In
everyday life it is easy to identify potentially stressful events
and experiences. This may relate to something very simple,

such as a train running late, to more extreme forms of stress, such as the death of a partner.

Stress has a number of origins:

- physical: e.g. exposure to heat, pain, exercise

- psychological: anxiety, fear, frustration

- social: bereavement or unemployment.

However, stress may also result from positive life events, such as holidays, weddings and Christmas.

The link between stress and disease was examined by Hans Seyle, who described the 'general adaptation syndrome'. Seyle defined stress as a non-specific psychobiological response of the body to any demand placed upon it to adapt. He observed that whether a situation was perceived positively or negatively, the physiological response of the body or arousal was similar; he argued that one cannot discriminate between good and bad stress. The 'general adaptation syndrome' is the process whereby the body tries to accommodate stress by adapting to it in a three-stage process. The three stages comprise:

> *Stage 1*: alarm reaction. The alarm reaction describes a 'fight-or-flight' response. In this stage several physiological responses occur. Initially this involves the nervous and the endocrine systems, followed by cardiovascular, pulmonary and muscoskeletal responses. The physiological responses to the alarm stage are summarised below.
> *Stage 2*: stage of resistance. The body tries to revert to a state of physiological calmness, or homeostasis, by the alarm. Because the perception of a threat still exists, however, complete homeostasis is never reached. Instead, the body stays activated or aroused, usually at a lesser intensity than during the alarm, but enough to cause a higher metabolic rate in some organs.

Stage 3: stage of exhaustion. Exhaustion occurs when one (or more) of the organs targeted by specific metabolic processes can no longer meet the demands placed upon it. The hormonal reserves are depleted, fatigue results and depression may be present. In its most extreme form this may lead to organ failure and death.

Seyle's general adaptation syndrome outlined the physiological consequences of stress. Through the activation of the hypothalamus, in the brain, there is stimulation of the pituitary gland, which is responsible for secreting several hormones. Adrenocorticotrophic hormone (ACTH) is the most significant in this context, as it stimulates the release of corticosteroids. This results in a variety of physiological effects; the most important is response to physical and psychological stress. The relationship between stress and disease involves several aetiological factors. These include the cognitive perceptions of the threatening stimuli and the consequent activation of the nervous, endocrine and immune systems.

The following are alarm reactions to fight-or-flight response:

- Release of adrenaline from adrenal medulla and glucocorticoid hormones from adrenal cortex resulting in:
    cardiovascular activity increases
    respiratory activity increases
    blood pressure rises
    muscles are toned
    pupils in the eyes become dilated
    gastrointestinal activity increases
    physiological sphincters of the body contract
    inflammatory response is suppressed

Bio-psychology reduces behaviour to its neural and biochemical elements. Study of the nerves and chemicals in the body to describe and explain behaviour has led to the development of a psychoneuroimmunological model of stress, defined as the intricate interaction of consciousness (psycho), brain and central nervous system (neuro), the body's defence against external infection and immunology.

The psychoneuroimmunological model of stress differs from that of Seyle. This model incorporates several distinct physiological responses to 'positive' and 'negative' stress. Thus stress may be interpreted as the inability to cope with a perceived or real threat to one's mental, physical, emotional, and spiritual well-being which results in a series of physiological responses and adaptations.

Life events and stress

One way of relating stress to illness has been to link it to life events. In the 1960s Holmes and Rahe developed the 'Social Readjustment Rating Scale' (SRRS), an inventory which ranks forty-three stressful events with numeric values, from most to least stressful, based upon their capacity to disrupt activities and the degree of readjustment which is necessary following an event. These values are termed 'Life Change Units' (LCU), a breakdown of which is listed in Table 3.1. They demonstrated that the development of minor illnesses, such as colds and flu, could be linked to life events.

Table 3.1 Measuring life stress: the life change scale

Life event	Life Change Units
Death of a spouse	100
Divorce	73
Marital separation	65
Marriage	50
Retirement	43
Vacation	13
Christmas	12

As this scale was devised over thirty years ago it is possible that changes in society have resulted in new or different stressors. Life-event scales have been criticised as indices of stress, due to their inability to differentiate the impact of positive as opposed to negative life events.

The life-event-scale approach also implies that individuals would respond in much the same way to similar situations, but the range of observed responses to these situations shows that individual differences may well be implicated in determining a stress reaction. Wide differences in both physiological and cognitive responses to stress are likely to be influenced by a variety of moderating variables, including personality and coping strategies.

Personality and stress

Personality in relation to stress has been classified by psychologists as either 'stress-prone' or 'stress-resistant' and individuals with these different characteristics may react very differently to similar stressful events. Type-A, co-dependency and helpless-hopeless are three personality sub-types that have been defined as being stress-prone.

Type-A individuals interpret any stressor as a threat to personal control and this seems to predispose these individuals to seek out demanding situations, consequently generating a great deal of stress for themselves. Type-B pattern of behaviour is less competitive and driven. The Type-A Behaviour Pattern (TABP) is characterised by striving for achievement, competitiveness and impatience. TABP may predispose to the development of ischaemic heart disease

Another influential factor in modulating the stress response is 'locus of control'. This concept arose from the observation that individuals give different reasons for events; the cause of an event could be external (e.g. luck) or internal (e.g. ability and effort) or a combination of the two. A person with an internal locus of control has an expectation that he or she will be able to control the environment, either through ability or effort. Someone with an external locus of control would tend to believe that outcomes are beyond personal control and depend on outside influences such as luck. Locus of control has been implicated in a wide range of health-related behaviours. In health care 'internals' are more likely to be proactive (i.e. eat healthily, smoke and drink less in order to reduce risk of heart disease). 'Externals' are more likely to think that ill-health won't happen to them, and if it does someone (i.e. a doctor or nurse) will take care of them. A sense of personal control over the environment is one of the principal components of the 'hardy' personality. A 'hardy' personality type is someone who in the face of disaster appears immune to stress. Having more internal control, or an internal locus of control, may serve as a buffer against stress. This personality is composed of three constructs:

1. willing to accept a challenge
2. commitment towards situations or events encountered
3. control and personal responsibility for life events.

Hardy individuals are viewed as mentally and physically healthier than others and have more effective coping strategies than non-hardy personality types. Some common coping strategies are listed in Table 3.2.

Coping

The ability to cope is a critical factor in adaptation to stressful life events. Coping has been defined as cognitive and behavioural efforts to manage specific external and/or internal demands that are appraised as taxing or exceeding the resources of the person. In order for a cognitive process to be considered as coping it must involve a purposeful effort. Adaptation can be seen as coming to terms with the reality of chronic illness, and includes letting go of false hope and hopelessness, as well as engaging in a process of restructuring the environment. Coping is a component or a 'subset' of adapting. It has been stated that 'the best coping is that which changes the person–environment relationship for the better'.

Coping styles may be involved in the response to stress and may be influenced by personality. Generally, coping can be viewed as a response to negative events, although the responses themselves are often defined in terms of stable traits.

Some researchers have speculated that the effect of a stressor may be buffered by an appropriate coping mechanism, and, to an extent, this view reflects popular belief. The supposed benefits of a 'good cry', or for that matter, a 'good laugh', are well known but it is less well understood what precisely constitutes an appropriate coping mechanism, and more importantly how to measure such a phenomenon.

Table 3.2 Maladaptive and adaptive coping

MALADAPTIVE COPING	ADAPTIVE COPING
Emotional	Detached
Feeling overpowered and helpless.	Not seeing situation or problem as a threat.
Becoming miserable, depressed and angry.	Keeping a sense of humour.
Taking frustrations out on others.	Seeing problem as separate from yourself.
Prepare for the worst possible outcome.	Resolve things by getting them into proportion.
Avoidance	Rational
Sitting tight and hoping it all goes away.	Use past experience to deal with situation.
Pretend there is nothing the matter.	Take action to change things.
Think about something else.	Take one step at a time, act logically.
Trust in fate: things will sort themselves out.	Give the situation full attention.

Social support

Social support is the perceived comfort that people derive from their social network. This includes partners, family, friends, community networks, church and health professionals.

It is believed that social support reduces the stress that people experience. Nurses should be aware that stress can have a detrimental effect on health, and social support can be protective against these adverse effects. Two theories have been generated to explain the protection provided by social support:

1. buffering hypothesis
2. direct-effect hypothesis.

The buffering hypothesis proposes that a good supportive network can buffer stress and the direct-effect hypothesis maintains that social support is beneficial, regardless of the amount of stress experienced.

Nurses are required to have an understanding of how stress can affect behaviour in order to understand the behaviour of patients. This allows the nurse to anticipate times when stress may be high and provide appropriate care.

PAIN

Very few of us will not have experienced the unpleasant physical sensation of pain at some point in our life. The pain which accompanies trauma such as burns, cuts or sprains represents a danger signal which prompts us to remove ourselves from the harmful situation and take action to protect the painful area. The management of pain is an integral part of the nursing role. Current understanding of pain recognises that it cannot be explained by purely physical means; it also requires an examination of psychological factors. An understanding of how psychological factors may influence pain makes a valuable contribution to good nursing care. This section examines psychological variables in relation to pain.

One of the most widely used and accepted nursing definitions of pain was provided by McCaffrey (1983); he suggested that pain is 'whatever the experiencing person says it is and existing whenever he says it does'. Nurses' knowledge and understanding of the mechanisms of pain and its relief are often left wanting. Research has shown that nurses often fail to

assess pain and pain relief systematically and that they often
tend to overestimate the pain relief obtained from analgesics
and underestimate the patient's pain.

Understanding pain

Pain is an unpleasant sensation which accompanies trauma or
disease. Despite the fact that pain is a universal experience,
there is no anatomical location for pain in the body. It is
believed that pain constitutes a complex interaction between
many peripheral and central neural structures and many areas
of the brain.

The physiology of pain

In most areas of the body physiological pathways include
nocicereceptors, the principal pain receptors. These are free
nerve endings of small myelinated A-delta fibres and the
unmyelinated C-fibres. These nocicereceptors are located
throughout the body. Somatic is the descriptor given to pain
that originates in the skin, muscles and joints. Visceral pain
describes that originating in the abdominal cavity or thorax.
Qualitatively the pain experience differs according to source.
The A-delta fibres are essentially somatic and transmit their
impulses very rapidly. This type of pain tends to be localised
and sharp in nature. The C-fibres can be deep somatic or
visceral and this impulse travels more slowly. This type of pain
tends to be more persistent, diffuse and aching in nature.
Sensory fibres are sensitive to a variety of stimuli, including
thermal, mechanical or chemical stimuli. They travel from the
site of origin and enter the spinal cord, where they synapse
with neurones (nerve cells).

The pain impulse results in the release of substance P,
considered to be the main neurotransmitter of pain. Substance
P allows the pain impulse to travel across the spinal cord and
connect with ascending pathways. There are several ascending

pathways for pain impulses. Impulses of the main tracts that have been identified ascend to the thalamus, in the brain, and relay on to the cerebral cortex. This activity allows the individual to make a perceptual discrimination as to the nature of the pain, to acknowledge it in order to respond to the pain and to make psychological evaluations of the pain.

Theories of pain

Both physiological and psychological processes contribute to the pain experience. The gate-control theory of pain was devised in the 1960s and provides the most comprehensive explanation of pain mechanisms. Melzack and Wall (1983) took the understanding of pain beyond that of sensations and demonstrated the importance of psychological processes on the pain experience. They hypothesised that the transmission of painful stimuli could be controlled by a gating mechanism and described descending pain-control mechanisms which could modulate or inhibit ascending pain signals. These inhibitory impulses may be under direct emotional and cognitive control in deciding how much pain the individual will feel. The gate theory provided insight into psychological influences on pain and added credibility to the use of psychological approaches to pain management, such as imagery and relaxation.

Beta-endorphins and enkephalins

As pain fibres enter the spinal cord, they may be subject to the inhibitory action of neurotransmitters, such as beta-endorphins and enkephalins. These are the human body's own natural opiate analgesics, receptor sites for which are found in the brain and spinal cord. Ekephalins play a peripheral role at neuronal synapses. In contrast, it is thought that beta-endorphins exert a central influence, modifying the painful experience via inhibitory descending pathways. Beta-endorphin release is under the control of the area of the cerebral cortex, which is also associated with emotions.

Therefore, it is possible to see how the psychological state may be directly associated with pain control. There is evidence that the cause and effect relationship may operate in both directions. Uncontrollable pain may trigger negative emotions, leaving an individual feeling anxious or depressed. Conversely, existing negative feelings may leave the pain gate open and reduce the individual's pain threshold. Nurses who appreciate this will realise that in aiming for pain relief, they are caring for the whole person and not just a physiological symptom.

Types of pain

The most important aspect for the nurse caring for someone in pain is believing that person's pain. However, in order for the nurse to assess the pain experience and plan an appropriate intervention, it is important to understand the differing types of pain that exist.

Acute and chronic pain

Acute pain can be differentiated from chronic pain on the basis of duration. Acute pain is usually sharp in nature, of relatively short duration and ends when the source is removed (e.g. the pain of kidney-stones is often very intense but immediately relieved upon passing them). Chronic pain is usually described as burning or aching in nature and lasts for a long period of time (e.g. chronic back pain). However, there are also psychological differences between acute and chronic pain. This relates to the cognitive and behavioural processes of adaptation which occur when an individual experiences persistent pain. Some types of pain, such as abdominal pain in irritable bowel syndrome, involve recurrent acute episodes of pain. Some individuals respond to, and manage, each episode of pain but remain fully functional in between. Others find that their lives are completely disrupted by the constant threat of a repeated attack of abdominal pain and these individuals become chronic pain sufferers.

Pain threshold and tolerance

Threshold refers to the intensity of stimulus necessary before a person perceives pain. Pain thresholds can be very high or even seemingly absent, for example, in situations of intense emotion. Conversely, chronic anxiety can reduce the pain threshold of an individual. Pain tolerance relates to the amount of pain that an individual is willing to endure before seeking relief. Tolerance can be increased through religious faith, culture, distraction and alcohol intake, whereas fear, anger, boredom and anxiety can reduce tolerance. Historically, Western society has looked favourably upon individuals who show a 'stiff upper lip' and 'grin and bear it', but these value judgements impair the capacity to help someone in pain.

Personality and pain

The personality of an individual can influence the experience of pain. Eysenck examined the relationship between specific traits of personality and pain responses. He was particularly interested in degrees of neuroticism and extraversion and demonstrated that anxiety, as part of the individual's unique personality structure, can have a negative effect on the pain experience.

The assessment of pain is covered in Chapter 4 under the section 'Clinical observations'.

WHAT IS SOCIOLOGY?

In contrast to disciplines such as biology and psychology, which focus on health at the individual level, sociology examines the social dimension of health, illness and health care. The role of sociology and its associated perspectives is to understand the social world that we live in. Once again the full range and complexity of sociological theory is beyond the remit of this text. It is, however, important for nurses to appreciate that sociological explanations of what it means to be a nurse or a patient owe much to the theoretical perspectives of sociologists.

It would be incorrect to say that there is a single sociological perspective or one correct sociological approach that is relevant to nurses. Sociology is characterised by a variety of perspectives that attempt to understand the social world in which we live. These perspectives range from those such as functionalism, which emphasises the value of social consensus and continuity, to those such as Marxism and political economy, which emphasise the sources of social conflict and change. Due to the brevity of this section readers are encouraged to refer to basic introductory sociology textbooks for additional information on these sociological perspectives. Sociology is the study of the structure of human society and how it functions. As individuals go about their everyday life there are two broad approaches that may be adopted. They may adopt a relatively passive approach, accepting rules, customs and laws in an unquestioning fashion. Alternatively, they may be actively involved in shaping events through arrangement and negotiation. These two contrasting approaches relate to two broad sociological perspectives, known respectively as structuralist and interpretative sociology. The structuralist sociologist views human beings as receivers of and responders to society, whereas the interpretative sociologist views them as manipulators and creators of social norms and rules.

Some familiarity with these two approaches may help potential nurses understand their role within the health-care setting and respect the social and cultural origins of their patients.

The sociological self is located in a variety of social and cultural contexts. It is involved in negotiating and constructing, with others, future roles in society. These interactive processes produce distinct individuals who interpret the culture in which they live in a unique way. Structuralism, as a broad approach, is based on the assumption that all of our social behaviour, attitudes and values are a result of the organisation and structure of the society in which we live. This approach focuses attention upon society as a set of interrelated, interdependent parts or systems, which include:

- the political system

- the legal system

- the economic system

- the medical system

- the educational system.

Within each of these systems a range of institutions and organisations exist. These control social relationships and actions, either in a compatible and harmonious fashion, or in a coercive or discordant manner. These two approaches are described by sociologist in terms of 'consensus' and 'conflict' sociology. Traditionally, the medical profession has enjoyed a significant amount of power. Doctors can sanction a number of social benefits such as patients' entitlement to health services and employees' sick leave. Consensus approaches accept the requirement of these functions for the smooth running of society. Indeed, the consensus approach suggests that because of their extensive training and commitment to ethical conduct those members of the regulated health professions (doctors and nurses) are well placed to carry out these functions. In contrast, conflict perspectives question professional power, highlighting issues of professional domination and social control, and the domineering impact of some of these practices.

Sociology and health

Sociology provides a number of distinctive and well-established approaches to questions about the social patterning of health and disease and the social impact of health-care intervention. These questions include:

- Do social structures, institutions and processes affect the health of individuals?

- What is the nature of the nurse–patient relationship?

- How does society make sense of health and illness?

- What impact do health-care services have on individuals and upon society?

- Are there social inequalities in health and illness?

Sociologists generally concentrate on causes of social division such as class, gender and ethnicity, which appear to have a powerful influence on society. For the purposes of this text these will be defined as:

- Class – the division and ranking of groups of people according to occupational role.

- Gender – the social meanings and values of the difference between the sexes. Gender refers to socially ascribed traits, characteristics and roles that are seen as belonging to either males or females.

- Ethnicity – the characteristics of social life, such as culture, language, history and religion, which are possessed by a group of people and passed on to the next generation.

One important area of study in sociology has been health-care institutions and their social context. Social factors, such as gender, have an important influence upon the make-up of various health professionals, in particular nursing.

As well as examining the social patterns of health and disease, sociologists are also concerned with social inequalities and their impact on health. Social inequalities can be defined as: inequalities in income; access to resources and power and status that is produced, reproduced and maintained by society. In order to measure inequalities people can be classified into five occupational categories ranging from social class I, which includes professional classes, to social class V, containing unskilled manual occupations. These classifications, although commonly used, are limited in a number of respects. Indeed, social classification does not accurately reflect the role of women in society, who traditionally are socially classified according to the occupation of male partners. The continued use of social classification is justified, for two reasons:

1. Occupation is the only socio-economic information recorded at census.
2. Occupation is regarded as a powerful determinant of income and life chances.

In the United Kingdom manual workers have consistently demonstrated poorer health and shorter life expectancy than their professional counterparts. Higher rates of illness and deaths consistently occur at earlier ages in individuals with poorer socio-economic circumstances.

Gender

The debate on gender and health relates to the anomaly that although women live longer than men do, they appear to have higher levels of poor health. Some diseases are sex specific, for example ovarian cancer in women and haemophilia in men. Lifestyle may also be associated with gender. Historically, males have consumed more alcohol and smoked more than females and undertaken more risky occupations and leisure activities. However, patterns appear to be changing and there is evidence to suggest that females are smoking and drinking more than ever before.

Biological explanations for the health differences between males and females focus upon the biological differences. Sociologists tend to reject the biological-based notions of gender identity and believe that social factors such as poor nutrition, and unequal access to health resources and reproductive risks make a significant impact on male-to-female mortality ratios. Sociologists make materialistic/structural explanations to examine health outcomes for men and women. This involves the examination of the varying social roles of men and women as well as differences in their access to resources such as income, employment, housing and leisure.

Ethnic group and health

Sociologists have generally rejected the notion that human groups can be unambiguously defined in terms of their genetic constitution. Social groups are more commonly defined by reference to a shared culture such as language, customs and institutions.

The sick role

Just as with other forms of behaviour, the way an individual behaves when he or she is ill is influenced by society. Being a patient implies that you are ill. Ill-health not only disturbs individual functioning, but can also be viewed as socially dysfunctional, undermining the values, activities and roles that contribute towards social stability.

Talcott Parsons (1975) developed the concept of the sick role to describe the expectations of people in a society that defines the rights and duties of its members who are sick. The sick role confers both rights and obligations.

The rights are:

- An exemption from responsibilities such as work and social obligations, which needs to be legitimised by a medical physician in order to be valid.

- That sick individuals avoid any blame or responsibility for their condition.

The two obligations are:

- The sick person must want to get better.

- The sick person must seek competent help, usually from a trained health professional.

Like many other roles in society, certain qualifications are required before the sick role can be taken up. First, the person must have a condition that has been defined by that culture to be a medical problem. Our society's views on what constitutes an illness have changed over time. For example, alcoholism is increasingly being viewed as a symptom of a disease rather than a sign of moral failure. Additionally, conditions such as HIV/AIDS carry some social stigma. This means that assumptions of responsibility and blame may influence how a person is seen and treated by others in society. The sick role gives a useful insight into the experience of illness and the role of medicine.

Defining health

The practice of nursing involves educating patients and promoting healthy lifestyles. Health promotion includes a wide range of strategies designed to improve people's health. Before health promotion can be examined it is important to first define health. Health is a broad concept that can embody a huge range of meanings, from the narrowly technical to the all-embracing moral and philosophical. When you think about your own health what is the answer to the following questions:

- I am healthy when . . . ?

- I am healthy because . . . ?

- To stay healthy I need . . . ?

- I become unhealthy when . . . ?

- My health improves when . . . ?

Health was defined by the World Health Organisation (WHO) as 'a state of complete physical, social and mental well-being, not merely the absence of disease or infirmity' (1985). It is important to appreciate that this definition moves away from a focus on the consequences of disease, highlighting people's social and mental health.

Disease, illness and ill-health

Disease, illness and ill-health are often used interchangeably. Disease is the objective state of ill-health; it is the existence of some pathology, or abnormality, of the body that is capable of detection. Illness is the subjective experience of loss of health. It is embedded in terms of symptoms, for example, the reporting of fever, pain, aches, or loss of function. Illness and disease are not the same, although there is a large degree of co-existence. For example, a patient may be diagnosed of having cancer through a screening programme even when they have had no symptoms. If a patient reports physical symptoms, and further investigations such as a blood test confirm a disease process, the two concepts of disease and illness coincide. It is in these situations that the term 'ill-health' can be used to refer to the experience of disease plus illness.

Health promotion

Health promotional activities may include preventive activities, education, community-based social action and the creation of healthy environments. Using these techniques people are encouraged to change their behaviour with respect to smoking, exercise, diet, safety, alcohol consumption, substance abuse and sexual activity. These techniques include a whole range of interventions including:

- Those that foster healthy lifestyles.

- Those that encourage access to services and involvement in health decisions.

- Those that seek to promote an environment in which the healthy choice becomes the easier choice.

- Those that educate about the body and keeping healthy.

In relation to nursing it has been shown that the process of health education often arises naturally in the interaction between nurses and patients. Health education is the process by which individuals and groups learn to promote, maintain or restore health. Its desired outcome is a change in behaviour or attitude, often in response to understanding the impact of the following factors on health:

- stress
- smoking

- exercise
- obesity

- chronic illness
- sexual activity.

Health education encourages people to take control of their own health; the knowledge it provides empowers them to make choices and decisions about themselves. Nurses may be involved in health-education programmes in a variety of settings, including hospitals, community health centres, shopping centres, clubs and schools. It is important that the health-promotion message must go beyond the individual and into society, influencing social policy and health-care plans. The role of the nurse in health promotion may involve one-to-one teaching, counselling, advising, and informing the public via publications, campaigns and community programmes.

Health promotion draws upon a variety of disciplines, including sociology, social psychology, education, economics, ethics and epidemiology, to inform its practice. It provides us with a way of looking at health that draws together all the factors that shape and influence the health of individuals and communities.

FURTHER READING

Beck, A. T., Rush, A. J., Shaw, B. F., and Emery, G. (1979) *Cognitive Therapy of Depression*, New York: John Wiley.

Birchenall, M. (1998), *Sociology as Applied to Nursing and Health Care*, London: Bailliere Tindall.

Erikson, E. (1965) *Childhood and Society*, Harmondsworth: Pelican.

Eysenck, H J (1967) *The Biological Basis of Personality*, Springfield, IL: C. C. Thomas.

Eysenck, H. J. (1970) *The Structure of Human Personality*, 3rd edn, London: Methuen.

Freud, S. (1976) [1900] *The Interpretation of Dreams*, Harmondsworth: Penguin.

McCaffrey, M. (1983) *Nursing the Patient in Pain*, London: Harper and Row.

Melzack, R., and Wall, P. D. (1983) *The Challenge of Pain*, New York: Basic Books.

Parsons, T. (1975) *The Social System*, New York: Free Press.

Payne, S., and Walker, J. (1997) *Psychology for Nurses and the Caring Professions*, Buckingham: Open University Press.

Rogers, C. R. (1961) *On Becoming a Person*, Boston: Houghton Mifflin.

4 AN INTRODUCTION TO CLINICAL SKILLS IN NURSING

It is the aim of this chapter to give nursing students the understanding to perform clinical observations accurately. It is hoped that this understanding will ensure that well-informed and accurate judgements are made about a patient's condition from observed results. Assessment of a patient's vital signs are basic nursing observations (temperature, pulse, respiration and blood pressure) and are often, although not always, taught at the beginning of nursing courses. It is important that student nurses can integrate the practice involved in these techniques with the biological science which gives them meaning. In this chapter, regular reference will be made to biological science material covered in Chapter 2 to facilitate this integration of knowledge. Vital signs provide an efficient and accurate method of monitoring a patient's condition and allow the nurse to evaluate any response to treatment and to detect problems at an early stage.

Specific observations covered in this section are:

• cardiovascular observations (pulse and blood pressure)

• respiratory observations

• body temperature

• eliminatory (digestive and urinary)

• neurological observations.

Before any nursing observations are recorded the nurse has a specific responsibility to adhere to the NMC guidelines concerning documentation and to be aware of local infection-control policies.

CARDIOVASCULAR OBSERVATIONS

The pulse

The alternate expansion and elastic recoil of an artery with each contraction of the heart is called the pulse. The pulse is caused by pressure being exerted by blood on the arterial wall, causing an expansion of the vessel for a brief moment as the wave of pressure passes. This pressure wave relates to the distension and recoil of the aorta, as blood leaves the left side of the heart. Consequently, the strongest pulse is present in the arteries which are closest to the heart. The pulse weakens as it passes through the arterial vessels, disappearing altogether by the time it reaches the capillary networks.

Assessment of a patient's pulse provides an efficient method of assessing the status of the heart and circulation.

All arteries demonstrate a pulse, but not all are accessible for nursing observation.

The pulse can be felt with fingers whenever an artery can be compressed gently against a bone. Recording the pulse with the thumb could lead to a false reading, as there is a weak pulse in the thumb. When measuring a pulse, it is important for the nurse to determine the rate, rhythm and amplitude or strength of the pulse beat.

For clinical purposes the pulse most commonly felt by nurses is the radial, where the radial artery passes over the radius. The radial pulse is found on the inner aspect of the wrist. The main advantages of using the radial pulse to monitor the pulse are:

• It is easy to access.

• It is not embarrassing for the patient.

- It is non-invasive.

- It is accurate.

While assessing the radial pulse of a patient, the nurse requires a watch with a second hand, a pen and the documentation sheet (TPR (temperature, pulse and respirations) chart) for recording the observation. It is important that prior to recording the pulse rate, the nurse explains the procedure to the patient.

The student nurse recording a radial pulse should:

- Ensure that the patient is lying or sitting down.

- Ensure that the patient has been at rest for a minimum of five minutes.

- Place the middle three fingers over the groove along the thumb side of the patient's wrist and press gently.

- If the pulse is regular the nurse should count the number of beats for thirty seconds and multiply the total number of beats by two.

- If the beat is irregular or has an abnormal strength of rhythm, the nurse should record the pulse for one full minute.

- Record the pulse rate on the TPR chart and report any abnormalities or changes in observation to a qualified nurse.

The radial pulse only loses accuracy when there is a drop in blood pressure. There are very few instances where the nurse will have difficulty locating a radial pulse, although patients with extremely obese arms often cause difficulties. Other areas include:

- brachial pulse: in the arm

- carotid pulse: in the neck

- femoral pulse: in the groin

- pedal pulse: in the foot

- popliteal pulse: behind the knee

- temporal pulse: at the side of the head.

Measurement of the pulse at these other sites is possible, but is associated with difficulties and should be reserved for specific circumstances. For example, the carotid pulse, which is situated in the neck, can be accessed in cardiac arrest. The nurse should only apply gentle pressure to this pulse, since the carotid artery provides blood supply to the brain and should not be occluded. The pedal pulses are important for the assessment of blood supply to the lower limbs. This form of assessment is particularly appropriate in the diagnosis of lower-limb vascular disease.

The radial pulse records the number of times the ventricles contract each minute; it is also possible to record this by listening to heart sounds with a stethoscope. This process is called auscultation and it involves counting the heart sounds per minute.

Many nurses involved in cardiac care are trained to observe heart sounds in this manner. It is important for them to listen for the ventricle at the outermost and lowest point of the heart, known as the apex beat. While listening for heart sounds the closure of the heart valves causes sounds, as the valve cusps vibrate. Several distinctive sounds can be heard: the first 'lubb' relates to the closure of the atrioventricular valves, and the second 'dubb' is the closure of the semi-lunar valves.

The pulse rate is equivalent to the number of heart beats per minute. Pulse rates may vary as a result of age, pain, anxiety, level of fitness, obesity, posture, temperature and a change in health status. To get an accurate assessment of the patient's condition, pain should be relieved, but the nurse should be aware of the implications of all these factors upon pulse rate.

Tachycardia is a fast pulse rate, which is usually defined as anything over 100 beats per minute. It is thought that the maximum heart rate possible is 180 beats per minute. Above this rate it is not possible for normal filling of the heart to take place. Tachycardia is often a feature of systemic infection.

Bradycardia is referred to as a slow heart rate, which it is usually defined as anything below 50 beats per minute. Bradycardia is often related to heart block. Heart block occurs when the impulses from the pacemaker in the heart, the sino-atrial (A) node, do not reach the ventricles and ventricular contraction rate slows down.

The strength of the pulse relates to two factors:

1. the stroke volume
2. the force applied to blood during ventricular contraction.

The electrocardiogram (ECG)

It is possible to measure the electrical activity in the heart using an instrument called an electrocardiogram (ECG). Electrodes are placed on the arms, legs and at six places across the chest and attached to the ECG. Each electrode records a slightly different electrical activity, because it is in a different position in relation to the heart. When electrical activity is measured three characteristic electrical phases can be seen. First, there is the P wave, followed by the QRS complex and T wave. The P wave occurs during atrial contraction, followed by QRS complex during ventricular contraction and finishing with the T wave, ventricular relaxation. A normal cardiac cycle has the PQRST phase in that order. The terms PQRST do not stand for anything and are just arbitrary letters given to the phases of electrical activity.

Blood pressure

Blood pressure in the body largely determined by the force exerted by blood on the walls of blood vessels. As described in Chapter 2, blood pressure varies in different blood vessels and also with the heart beat.

Blood circulates due to the pressure gradient that the heart establishes. The highest average pressure is created by the left ventricular pump, in the aortic arch, and the lowest pressure in the junction between the inferior and superior vena cavae.

Unless otherwise stated in this section, the term 'blood pressure' refers to blood pressure in the large arteries.

Maintenance of blood pressure is fundamental to the perfusion of blood through all body tissues. Examples of this are the lungs, which need a constant supply of blood for gas exchange, the kidneys which must have adequate blood pressure to maintain filtration of urine, and the digestive system which requires blood to collect nutrients from food. Therefore, blood pressure is an index of many of the physiological processes in the body, and the student nurse should understand the necessity for its measurement in clinical practice.

Physiology of blood pressure

Systemic arterial blood pressure is caused by the contraction of the left ventricle and the resistance to flow within the circulation.

When measuring the blood pressure two readings are recorded. The higher value is the systolic pressure and the lower value is the diastolic pressure.

During systole (ventricular contraction), the left ventricular myocardium pushes blood into the aorta, and this surge of blood causes the artery to distend. This wave of high pressure is then generated through the arterial system to the capillary network, reaching its lowest value in the venous return to the heart.

The diastolic pressure is the pressure in the arteries when the heart is in diastole, when the ventricles relax.

Resistance to flow is created by peripheral resistance. Peripheral resistance is the resistance offered by blood vessels to the flow of blood. In the circulatory system this is achieved first by the reduction in size of the arterioles into smaller vessels, and then by a process of vasoconstriction and vasodilation.

Vasoconstriction = decrease in diameter of lumen of a
vessel
Vasodilation = increase in diameter of lumen of a vessel

Involuntary smooth muscles in the walls of vessels make these changes to the lumen diameter in response to the sympathetic nervous system. This is influenced by a region in the medulla of the brain, the vasomotor centre (VMC). This centre has a profound effect upon blood pressure as it can initiate variations in the peripheral resistance by adjusting the vasoconstrictor tone. To perform this role the VMC receives feedback from baroreceptors, pressure receptors, based in the arch of aorta and carotid arteries, which directly measure blood pressure and relate the information back to the centre. This is a good example of a homeostatic negative feedback system. Normal blood pressure is therefore maintained by an average vasoconstrictor tone stimulation from the control centre.

Local factors which may influence blood pressure are temperature and physical trauma, such as burns.

Blood pressure can therefore be viewed as a combination of many effects; the output from the heart (the cardiac output) and the peripheral resistance in the circulation. This can be expressed in the following way:

Blood pressure = cardiac output (heart rate × stroke volume) × peripheral resistance

The average normal blood pressure for a young adult is 120/80mmHg and for an older adult 140/90mmHg.

Observation of blood pressure
The student nurse recording a blood pressure will require a

stethoscope, a sphygmomanometer with an appropriate sized cuff, a pen and the documentation sheet (TPR chart) for recording the observation. It is important that prior to recording the blood pressure the nurse explains the procedure to the patient and emphasises the need to refrain from speaking while the blood pressure is being measured, since this may lead to a false reading.

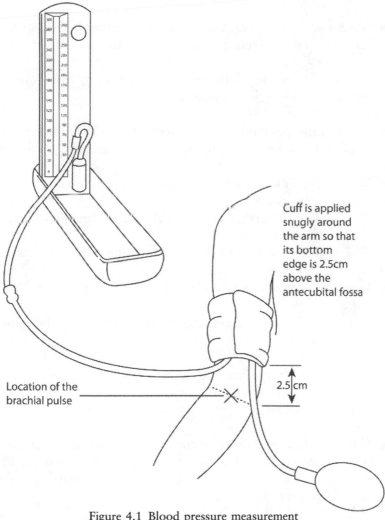

Cuff is applied snugly around the arm so that its bottom edge is 2.5cm above the antecubital fossa

Location of the brachial pulse

2.5 cm

Figure 4.1 Blood pressure measurement

The student nurse should then:

- Get the patient to sit or lie down.

- Ensure the patient is comfortable.

- Ensure the patient has not eaten or drunk alcohol or caffeine in the previous thirty minutes.

- Select the arm for cuff placement, avoid the following: an arm with an intravenous cannula; side of mastectomy.

- Remove restrictive clothing from the chosen arm (obese patients may require a larger cuff).

- Position the patient's arm horizontally, so that the cuff is level with the heart and palm is facing upwards.

- Palpate the brachial artery (in the bend of the arm).

- Position the cuff so that the centre is over the brachial artery.

- Wrap the deflated cuff evenly around the patient's arm.

- Position the manometer on level surface at eye level.

- Palpate the brachial artery and position stethoscope beneath the cuff.

- Inflate the cuff to 30mmHg above the point that pulsation disappears (cuff should be inflated quickly to prevent venous congestion).

- Slowly deflate the cuff, noting the pressure at which the pulse reappears. (This is systolic blood pressure (Korotkoff sounds).) The sound of blood flow can be heard in five distinct phases, see Table 4.1 below.

- Fully deflate the cuff, noting where the sound disappears. (This is the level of diastolic blood pressure.)

- Record blood pressure on TPR observation chart.

- If the procedure has to be repeated, allow a brief pause to allow blood to flow to and from arm.

- Reassure patient at end of measurement.

- Inform trained nursing staff of any abnormalities in recording.

It is important to follow these procedures correctly, including keeping the arm straight and supported, to maintain accuracy.

Table 4.1 Korotkoff sounds and phases

Phase	Sound
I	Appearance of tapping sounds that increase in intensity.
II	Softening of sounds that may become swishing.
Auscultatory gap	Sounds disappear for short time.
III	Return of sharper sounds, to level of Phase I.
IV	Distinct, abrupt muffling of sounds, which becomes soft.
V	The point at which all sounds disappear.

Avoiding errors measuring blood pressure
There are several factors which lead to errors when recording a patient's blood pressure. These problems can relate to the nurse, the patient or the equipment. Student nurses should never take a guess at the pressure. If they have a difficulty hearing Korotkoff sounds they should report it to a qualified member of the nursing staff. It is far better to own up to being unable to record a patient's blood pressure than to place the patient in jeopardy with a false reading.

There are many factors which can lead to the recording of a misleading blood pressure in patients. If patients are too warm or cold, anxious or in pain, their blood pressure will be affected. Nurses should also be aware of how to check the equipment used to measure blood pressure. The following factors are common sources of error:

- Mercury has not been set to zero in the manometer.

- Numbers on the manometer are not clearly visible.

- Equipment may not be correctly calibrated.

- There may be defective control valves or flaws in the cuff.

Abnormalities in blood pressure
Abnormalities of systolic blood pressure either relate to hypertension or hypotension. These terms can be defined as:

- Hypertension – blood pressure is raised above normal value for patient's age or condition.

- Hypotension – blood pressure is lower than normal values.

An approximate guide to what is high or low is the pressure 100mmHg. If diastolic rises above 100mmHg this suggests hypertension, but if systolic drops below 100mmHg this suggests hypotension.

High blood pressure
Blood pressure usually rises with age, but hypertension produces symptoms resulting in damage to organs and tissues, especially related to the heart and blood vessels.
A high blood pressure is a systolic pressure of 160–180mmHg and above. The diastolic pressure is also raised as a general rule; a high diastolic pressure is usually in the region of 90–120mmHg or above. Malignant hypertension is regarded as diastolic pressure exceeding 130mmHg. The result of persistent hypertension can be the combination of several complications. These include:

- Rupture of a blood vessel, in particular in the brain, which is one of the causes of cerebrovascular accident and stroke.

- Enlargement of the heart, known as cardiac hypertrophy, which can lead to cardiac failure.

- Arteriosclerosis, or hardening of the arteries, which is due to changes in the blood vessel walls.

Common risk factors for developing hypertension are:

- increasing age

- obesity

- high levels of salt in the diet

- smoking

- family history of hypertension

From the nursing perspective it is important to note that many of the risk factors are controllable by the patient. The nurse as a health educator can advise individuals to reduce their risk of hypertension by not smoking, reducing their weight and reducing salt intake.

Low blood pressure
As previously stated, a low blood pressure is a systolic pressure of less than 100mmHg. Low blood pressure can result from haemorrhage, physiological shock and heart failure. The danger with low blood pressure relates to the insufficient supply of oxygenated blood to vital areas, such as the brain. Low blood pressure is strongly resisted by the body's compensatory mechanisms, which strive to increase blood pressure. This is achieved through vasoconstriction of arterioles to increase peripheral resistance, plus an increase in heart rate to increase cardiac output.

Some hormones, for example adrenaline and noradrenaline, act as short-term homeostatic regulators of low blood pressure by increasing cardiac output. Other hormones are longer-term regulators, which act by influencing the volume of blood in the body and peripheral resistance; these include aldosterone and anti-diuretic hormone.

The ultimate extreme of hypotension is termed 'shock'. This occurs when the body's compensatory mechanisms fail to maintain the blood pressure. Hypovolaemic shock can result from massive bleeding, which can be internal (e.g. gastrointestinal bleed) or external (into the outside environment, e.g. following a road traffic accident).

Specific nursing care of the patient with low blood pressure includes:

- Ensuring the patient is flat with the foot of the bed raised.

- Giving heart stimulants, such as adrenaline, to stimulate circulation and cause vasoconstriction to peripheral blood vessels.

- Increasing fluids in the circulation, such as saline, by intravenous infusion or a blood transfusion.

RESPIRATORY OBSERVATIONS

Normal breathing is regular and rhythmic. Respiratory values vary with age, gender and medical presentation. On average the normal breathing rate of a healthy adult is 12–20 breaths per minute. When a nurse is observing a patient's respiratory rate, rhythm and depth it is advisable not to let the patient know as people tend to breathe differently if they know they are being observed. Student nurses are recommended to measure respiratory rate immediately after they have recorded the pulse rate.

Chest movement should be equal, bilateral and symmetrical in normal breathing.

The most sensitive indicator of respiratory distress is a rise in an individual's respiratory rate. As normal breathing is barely audible it is commonplace to use a stethoscope to listen for lung sounds. The following signs are an indication of respiratory distress:

- Noisy respiration is a sign of respiratory distress.

- A 'wheeze' is characteristic of asthma or bronchitis.

- A 'rattly' noise indicates the presence of fluid in the respiratory tract.

BODY TEMPERATURE

Core body temperature is controlled by the hypothalamus in the base of the brain. The hypothalamus acts as a homeostatic negative feedback mechanism. If the body temperature rises, mechanisms come into action, so that heat is lost from the body. Conversely, if the body temperature falls, heat is conserved until normal body temperature is restored. At 37°C, the human body temperature is well balanced to provide optimal condition for metabolic reactions in the body. Usually, body temperature remains relatively stable, fluctuating only 0.5°C from the normal.

Nurses measure body temperature for two important reasons:

1. To provide insight into the metabolic and homeostatic activity of the body.
2. To provide information about the possible causes of an abnormal health state.

It is important for the nurse to be aware of the many factors which can influence body temperature. These include:

- prolonged exposure to a hot or cold environment

- exercise

- hormonal disturbances

- altered white-cell count

- trauma (e.g. burns)

- infection

- damage to the hypothalamus

- reaction to blood products.

Core temperature is the temperature within the core of the body, in the main organs. Peripheral temperature is the temperature on the surface of the skin or in the hands and feet. Normally, there is a 1°C difference between the core and peripheral temperatures, but this difference can increase in extremely cold conditions by as much as 10°C.

The basic physiology of heat regulation in the body is introduced in Chapter 2.

Heat production is part of the energy obtained from cellular metabolism of adenosine triphosphate (ATP), a high-energy molecule. Enzymes within the mitochondria of a cell produce ATP from the metabolism of nutrients.

Removal of heat from the body occurs mainly through the skin. Sweating is an indicator that the body is too hot and a means by which heat is lost. Sweating is an example of evaporation of heat from the body. Other means of skin heat loss are convection, conduction and radiation:

- *Convection* – warming of air next to skin

- *Conduction* – passage of heat from skin on to cooler objects

- *Radiation* – transfer of heat from one object to another without touch.

Heat is also lost in faeces, urine and exhaled air, which is warmed in the respiratory tract. It is not surprising that with all these forms of heat loss from the body a cold room full of people can very quickly heat up.

These cooling mechanisms only work within a limited range. If the environment gets too hot or heat-loss mechanisms are inhibited, then body temperature will rise and hyperthermia will develop. Hyperthermia does not become a major problem up to a temperature of 40°C. However, at temperatures above 40°C the brain has a reduced ability to function normally and if the temperature reaches 45°C death from hyperthermia can result.

If our body temperature falls we can perform behavioural changes such as shivering or arterial vasoconstriction (to minimise heat loss). In order to conserve heat, the superficial veins will also constrict. The hair erector muscles will contract, causing hair to 'stand on end'. This allows for the conservation of heat by increasing the insulation of the body.

Hypothermia

Hypothemia results from general loss of body heat from exposure to a cold environment. It can occur at any age, but by far the largest number of cases occur in the very young and the very old. If core body temperature drops below 35°C, this may be described as hypothermia. In a cold environment our heat-gain mechanisms can fail and result in a drop in body temperature. A drop in temperature has several effects on the body including a reduced metabolic function. If hypothermia is suspected the nurse should use a low-reading thermometer.

The body has the ability to switch from increased heat production when it is cold to increased heat loss when it is hot. This is a finely tuned homeostatic process that is very sensitive to the smallest of changes in internal and external temperature. The aim of this homeostatic mechanism is to stabilise body temperature at an average of 37°C; this process is called normothermia. Body temperature is therefore a balance between heat gained and heat lost. Other terms that the student nurse may encounter related to body temperature are:

• pyrexia fever: temperature above normal value

• afebrile: without a fever.

Measurement of body temperature

Nurses can assess body temperature at a variety of sites in the body. Average normal temperature varies according to the measurement site used. The average temperature readings for adults are as follows:

• oral temperature (in mouth) 37°C

• rectal temperature (in rectum) 37.5°C

• axilla temperature (under armpit) 36.5°C

• tympanic temperature (in ear) 36.8°C–37.9°C.

Historically, mercury thermometers were the only type of thermometer used by nurses to measure temperature. However, these have been phased out and disposable, electronic and infrared thermometers are gaining wider clinical use. The main reason for this change relates to the risks associated with the breakage of glass, mercury poisoning and risks of cross-infection encountered with glass mercury thermometers. Electronic and infrared thermometers have also been shown to be quicker and to provide more accurate readings. Electronic devices are available to measure oral, axillary and rectal temperatures. Infrared thermometers are primarily for use in the ear, measuring the temperature in the tympanic membrane in a matter of seconds (see Figure 4.2). As the ear drum shares the same blood supply as the hypothalamus, tympanic readings are very close to core body temperature.

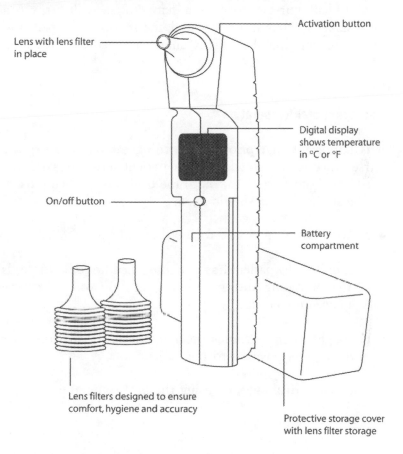

Activation button

Lens with lens filter in place

Digital display shows temperature in °C or °F

On/off button

Battery compartment

Lens filters designed to ensure comfort, hygiene and accuracy

Protective storage cover with lens filter storage

Figure 4.2 Tympanic membrane thermometer

Disposable thermometers are also available and they have been shown to be less expensive and just as efficient as electronic thermometers. They comprise a series of temperature-sensitive chemical colour dots to provide an easily read system.

Observation of body temperature

The student nurse recording a temperature will require a disposable, electronic or infrared thermometer, a pen and the documentation sheet (TPR chart) for recording the temperature.

Measuring oral temperature

It is important that prior to recording the temperature the nurse explains the procedure to the patient and emphasises the need to refrain from speaking if the oral route is being used. The student nurse should then:

● Assess whether it is safe to use the oral site.

● Ensure that the patient has not consumed hot or cold fluids in the preceding fifteen minutes, as this will affect the temperature recorded.

● Highlight the importance of maintaining the thermometer in the correct position to the patient.

The main advantages of using the oral route are:

● It is easily accessible.

● Its close proximity to the carotid artery allows measurement of the core temperature.

Measuring rectal temperature

Although it is potentially uncomfortable and embarrassing for patients, the rectal site does provide a safe location for measurement of temperature. It is used primarily for the measurement of temperature in the unconscious patient and requires the use of a specific rectal thermometer (usually marked with a blue tip). The recent development of use of tympanic (ear) thermometers in clinical areas has seen a reduction in the need for using the rectum for temperature measurement.

Measuring tympanic (ear) temperature

Tympanic temperature provides an accurate core reading because of the ear's close proximity to the hypothalamus.
   The student nurse should:

- Ensure that patient removes hearing aids.

- Prepare the tympanic thermometer.

- Place disposable ear cover.

- Insert probe into the ear.

- Hold the thermometer in the ear until a reading is displayed on unit.

- Dispose of probe cover.

- Inform patient of reading.

- Document measurement and indicate that the tympanic site was used.

- Report any abnormalities or changes to qualified nursing staff.

ELIMINATION: URINARY OBSERVATIONS

The main components of the urinary system are the kidneys. They act to remove metabolic wastes from the blood by forming them into urine. Urine is passed from the kidneys through the ureters to the urinary bladder, where it is stored. Besides removing waste products from tissue cells, the kidneys maintain the volume of water in the blood and regulate salt concentration and pH of blood. The urinary system therefore plays an important role in the homeostasis of the body, maintaining constant conditions within the tissue fluids of the cells.

The nurse should be familiar with normal and abnormal states of urine production. Although urine is a waste product of the body, it can offer a unique insight into the physiological workings of many of the body systems. Through accurate observation of urine nurses can reveal much about their patients.

There are several basic observations that nurses can make with a sample of urine:

- note the smell

- note the volume

- note the colour

- note the presence of deposits

- test for specific gravity.

There are a number of terms and abbreviations that student nurses may encounter in relation to the urinary system that they may not be familiar with. Some examples include:

- PU: passing urine

- UTI: urinary tract infection

- HNPU: has not passed urine

- micturition: the act of passing urine

- voiding: emptying the bladder

- + plus sign indicating the amount of urine passed (+++ = a lot)

- haematuria: presence of blood in the urine.

When should nurses test urine?

Most tests of urine are quick, cheap, non-invasive with on-the-spot results. Other tests require laboratory analysis, which is time consuming, more expensive and usually takes days for results.

Types of urine samples include:

- urinalysis

- early-morning urine samples (EMU)

- 24-hour urine collection

- midstream specimen of urine (MSU)

- catheter sample of urine.

Urinalysis

The term 'urinalysis' refers to the testing of urine for a variety of solutes. Eight separate tests have been incorporated to measure amounts of important solutes in urine that may be indicative of a disease process. Urinalysis provides the nurse with an immediate wealth of information concerning the patient's kidneys, urinary tract and liver as well as important information concerning metabolic and endocrine functions.

The student nurse performing urinalysis will require a

reagent strip and a bottle, a receiver, a watch with a second hand, gloves, pen and result sheet to record the urinalysis.
The student nurse should then:

- Take urine sample to sluice/investigation area.

- Remove a reagent strip from bottle (check that this is not out of date).

- Immerse all the reagent stick in the urine sample (ensure all pads are covered).

- Note position of second hand on watch.

- Hold strip horizontally to prevent mixing of reagent chemicals.

- At stated time compare reagent stick with corresponding chart on bottle.

- Make a note of the urinalysis results on results sheet.

- Discard urine and place reagent stick in clinical waste bin.

- Remove gloves and wash hands.

- Inform qualified nursing staff of result if significant.

It should be noted that NAD is clinical shorthand for 'nothing abnormal detected' and is often used to record findings.
Urinalysis or urine reagent sticks usually test urine for:

- protein

- glucose

- blood

- ketones

- bilirubin

- urobilinogen

- haemoglobin

- pH (normal range for urine 4.5–8.0).

Abnormal findings

Protein does not normally appear in the urine. Blood proteins albumin, globulin, fibrinogen and prothrombin are usually too large to pass through the glomerular membrane pores. Protein in the urine, termed proteinuria, can be indicative of damage or infection of kidney tissue.

Glucose is usually filtered via the glomerulus and then absorbed back into the blood. Under normal circumstances the return of glucose into the blood system is total, leaving no glucose in either the filtrate or the urine. Presence of glucose in the urine is indicative of diabetes mellitis.

Blood in the urine, haematuria, is perfectly normal in some circumstances (e.g. during menstruation, after bladder surgery). However, it is often indicative of pathophysiology and requires investigation. Blood in the urine can be the result of trauma (e.g. a tumour) to any part of the renal system, or be present during infection.

Ketones
Ketones are the end product of the breakdown of fat in the body. These may be excreted in urine or may be reused for energy in the body. High levels of ketones in the urine may indicate that a patient has not been eating or has diabetes mellitis. Presence of ketones will give urine a distinctive sweet, pear-drop smell.

Bilirubin and urobilinogen
Bilirubin and urobilinogen are products of haemoglobin breakdown when it is released from destroyed red cells. Increased levels of these solutes are indicative of liver or biliary disease. Both bilirubin and urobilinogen are not normally found in the urine and their presence makes urine very dark. These levels are commonly raised in jaundice.

Other solutes that can be present in urine that have clinical significance are:

• Nitrites – usually indicative of infection in the urine.

• Leucocytes – usually indicative of inflammation and infection.

At present nitrite and white-blood-cell tests are laboratory based and patients are often required to wait for several days for results; scientists are trying to incorporate these tests on to a reagent strip.

Specific gravity
The density of urine identifies how much solute there is present. Specific gravity is the weight of a known volume of liquid divided by the weight of an equal volume of pure water. Therefore, the specific gravity of urine is a measure of the urine's density compared to the density of pure water. The normal range of specific gravity of urine is 1010–1030. This value is affected by both water concentration and solute concentration in the urine.

Urine is also routinely pH as an acid–alkali measurement of urine. In urine the hydrogen ion (pH) concentration varies according to diet and tissue metabolism. The normal pH of urine varies from pH 5 to 8. Increased urinary pH (>pH 8) occurs in alkolosis and low urinary pH (<pH 5) appears in acidosis.

Early morning urine (EMU) is a sample collected first thing in the morning. The first voided urine is usually the most concentrated and is the preferred specimen when testing for substances which have a low concentration in the body, for example for hormones in pregnancy tests.

A 24-hour urine collection can be used to assess the amount of a substance that is lost in the urine. It may be collected at home or within the hospital. All urine must be saved throughout a 24-hour period. For example, the creatinine clearance test measures amounts of creatinine in a 24-hour period. Increased levels are indicative of advanced renal disease.

With a midstream specimen (MSU) of urine, the objective is to collect a sample that is uncontaminated by bacteria. MSU specimens are usually required for microscopy, culture and sensitivity when a urinary tract infection is suspected.

Patients who have a urinary catheter inserted as part of their care are at higher risk of developing a catheter-related infection as:

- There is an obstruction to the normal closing of the bladder by the catheter.

- There is a loss of the natural flushing of the urethra by passing urine.

- There is a risk of urinary backflow if catheter becomes kinked.

A catheter sample of urine (CSU) is usually taken as an aseptic technique. Aseptic technique is a method of carrying out a procedure in an environment that is rendered as free from micro-organisms as possible.

The formation of urine is covered in Chapter 2.

ELIMINATION: DIGESTIVE OBSERVATIONS

The digestive system consists of all the organs involved in the ingestion, digestion and absorption of food and in the elimination from the body of undigested food. The structure and basic functions of the gastrointestinal tract are covered in Chapter 2.

Essentially, the gastrointestinal tract is a single muscular tube that runs from the mouth to the anus. The accessory organs, liver, gall bladder and pancreas are not part of the gastrointestinal tract; however, as they secrete digestive enzymes they are extremely influential in the digestive process.

Abnormal elimination from the digestive tract, such as diarrhoea or vomiting, is often viewed as unpleasant or distasteful. However, the nurse should be aware of any abnormality or change in pattern of elimination, as it is an indication that physiological changes have occurred in the gastrointestinal tract. Alteration in the usual pattern of elimination can be related to a variety of factors including:

- infection of the gut (e.g. gastroenteritis)

- medication (e.g. antibiotic therapy can result in diarrhoea)

- reduced mobility can result in constipation

- dietary factors (insufficient fruit and fibre may result in constipation)

- emotional disturbances (anxiety can lead to diarrhoea)

- a disease in another body part (thyroid disease can give diarrhoea).

Observation of the products of elimination is an important nursing role and an understanding of the facts gained from observation, combined with a knowledge of underlying disease processes, allows nurses greater opportunities to make well-informed decisions for their patients.

There are a number of terms and abbreviations that student nurses may encounter in relation to elimination that they may not be familiar with. Some examples include:

- defaecation: opening of the bowels

- emesis: vomiting

- haematemesis: vomiting blood

- stools: faeces

- melaena: dark tarry stool, indicating bleed in GI tract

- BO: bowels open

- BNO: bowels not open

- straining: trying hard to pass faeces

- + plus sign indicating the amount of stool passed (+++ = a lot).

Diarrhoea

This results when movements of the intestine occur too rapidly for water to be absorbed in the colon. Stools are consequently produced in large amounts and may range from being loose to being entirely liquid, such as the 'rice water' stools associated with cholera. Diarrhoea, depending on its severity and duration, can be a mere nuisance or can be fatal. If diarrhoea is severe, large amounts of water (consisting of ingested fluids and digestive juices, together with sodium and potassium) are lost in the stools. This rapidly results in dehydration and electrolyte imbalance. Children with diarrhoea and vomiting can quickly become severely dehydrated.

The patient with diarrhoea may be exhausted, have abdominal pain, be possibly embarrassed, be anxious and have excoriation of the perineum. Nursing activities should be directed towards the relief of these problems.

Causes of diarrhoea are the following:

- *Diet*: certain foods, notably fruits and highly seasoned dishes, can result in diarrhoea.

- *Drugs*: certain drugs, for example antibiotics and iron preparations, cause diarrhoea in some people. Laxatives, by definition, result in the passage of a large, loose stool.

- *Infections*: organisms such as *salmonella* and *E. Coli* (*Escherichia coli*) can produce an inflammatory enteritis when present in sufficient numbers. Such intestinal infections are commonly accompanied by nausea and abdominal pain and usually follow the ingestion of contaminated food.

- *Inflammatory conditions of the gastrointestinal tract*: these include, for example, ulcerative colitis, irritable bowel syndrome and regional ileitis (Crohn's disease).

- *Malabsorption syndrome*: in conditions in which food is not absorbed from the ileum, bulky, offensive stools can be produced.

- *Tumours*: malignant growths in the bowel may result in a change of bowel habits, such as alternating periods of diarrhoea and constipation.

- *Stress*: diarrhoea may be a physiological response to stress.

In treating diarrhoea, the predisposing cause must be sought and treated and dehydration and electrolyte imbalances must be corrected. Concurrently, provision should be made for the symptomatic relief of the problems presented to the patient by the condition, for example the position of an inpatient's bed in the ward must be carefully considered. If the patient is ambulant, it is helpful if his or her bed is situated not too far from the lavatory. If the patient is on bedrest, then provision must be made for adequate ventilation of the bed area and for deodorant sprays. Soft lavatory paper or tissues are most comfortable for the patient, and sometimes a barrier cream for the perineal area is helpful to prevent excoriation. Diarrhoea is an unpleasant condition which causes many patients embarrassment and worry, so reassurance that they are not a nuisance is frequently necessary.

Constipation

This term refers to the difficult passage of hard stools. Many people may wrongly regard themselves as being constipated if they do not defaecate every day. However, it may be normal for one person to have two bowel actions every day whereas for another it is normal to defaecate only two or three times each week. In this latter case, so long as the stools are of normal consistency and are not difficult to pass, such a person could not be regarded as being constipated.

Constipation is the opposite of diarrhoea in that the food residues become hard due to the reabsorption of most of the water when they remain in the colon for a long time. They thus become difficult and often painful to eliminate. Constipation frequently occurs when the diet contains insufficient fibre. Constipation usually results in the patient complaining of a feeling of fullness or of feeling 'bloated'. Additionally, halitosis, a furred tongue, headache, irritability and flatulence may also occur with constipation. Haemorrhoids further serve to aggravate the problem of constipation as the sufferer tends to delay defaecation in an attempt to avoid the consequent pain.

Causes of constipation are the following:

- *Avoidance of defaecation*: the embarrassment of having to use a bedpan or commode in the close vicinity of other patients may lead to constipation in any patient in hospital. At home, the patient who is too weak or who is in too much pain (for example, from arthritis) to move to the lavatory may avoid defaecation.

- *Dehydration*: a decrease in fluid intake, or an increase in fluid loss, can cause constipation.

- *Depression and dementia*: both of these conditions result in a general slowing down of both physical and mental activities. This would include the slowing down of colonic movements and constipation may result. Antidepressant drug therapy may further serve to worsen the condition.

- *Drugs*: certain analgesics, notably codeine, and iron preparations may all cause constipation, and sufferers may attempt to avoid the passage of stools.

- *Inactivity*: exercise tends to stimulate peristalsis and thus defaecation. Patients who are on prolonged bedrest may therefore suffer from constipation.

- *Insufficient dietary fibre*: dietary fibre is hygroscopic (i.e. attracts water). It therefore provides bulk to the stool and aids elimination. Elderly patients without their own teeth or with badly fitting dentures may tend to eat a soft, low-fibre diet, and thus aggravate the problems arising from weak musculature of the pelvic floor.

Complications of constipation

In order to initiate the call to stool, a faecal mass of 100–150g is necessary. If the faecal mass is less than this, then straining is necessary in order to eliminate it. During straining, momentary circulatory stasis occurs, with an increase in blood pressure. The increase in blood pressure can result in the rupture of an existing aneurysm in the cerebral circulation or aorta.

It should be possible to prevent constipation by increasing the intake of dietary fibre to 30g a day and by encouraging an adequate amount of exercise. People eating a high-fibre diet should increase their fluid intake in order to prevent its hygroscopic action leading to dehydration.

Management of constipation

The student nurse should be aware that the position the patient adopts for defaecation affects the efficiency of the mechanism. A comfortable squatting position is more efficient than an upright one. Sitting on a bedpan is uncomfortable and consequently does not aid defaecation; it may in fact increase the amount of straining required.

The administration of oral or rectal lubricants, such as liquid paraffin orally, or glycerine suppositories rectally, serves to soften the faeces. The commonest bowel stimulants (aperients) are the senna derivatives, bisacodyl and Senokot. It is thought that these substances irritate the colonic mucosa and thus aid defaecation. Examples of osmotic aperients are Epsom salts, which can be given either orally or as an enema, oral milk of magnesia and phosphate enemas. These substances are hygroscopic, that is, they draw water into the lumen of the gut from the surrounding blood capillaries. A large watery stool will therefore follow their administration.

Bulking agents, such as dietary fibre and Movicol, reduce mouth-to-anus transit time by attracting water to the gut contents and thus providing a bulky but relatively soft stool.

If the above methods fail to manage the problem of constipation, then in extreme circumstances it may be necessary to carry out a manual removal of faeces. This is a painful and embarrassing procedure and should only be attempted by a trained nurse experienced in the technique.

Assessment of the patient's normal elimination habits is of vital importance. As highlighted above, elimination patterns are affected by many factors and each individual will have his or her own 'normal' toileting habit.

A healthy adult usually eliminates 100–150g of faeces per day. This consists of water (approximately 70–100g) and solids (30–50g). The solids are made up of indigested food, cellulose, epithelial cells from the lining of the digestive tract, some salts and a brown-coloured pigment stercobilin. The distinctive brown colour of stools results from the breakdown of bile.

Faecal samples

The most common observations that nurses are required to make of a faecal sample are:

- colour

- frequency

- amount

- consistency

- odour

- presence of foreign substances

- any pain or discomfort on defaecation.

Vomiting

This occurs as a result of a reflex and can be defined as the forceful expulsion of gastric and intestinal contents through the mouth. During the process the larynx is closed and the soft palate rises to close off the nasophrynx and so prevent the inhalation of vomitus. The diaphragm and abdominal wall contract strongly, the pylorus closes and this results in a sharp rise in the intragastric pressure, which causes the sudden expulsion of the gastric contents.

The vomiting centre is situated in the medulla oblongata of the brain. Impulses travel from the vomiting centre to the muscles of the abdominal wall and diaphragm via the extra-pyramidal tract, and to the stomach via the vagus nerve.

Vomiting may be stimulated by any of the following:

- Irritation of any part of the gastrointestinal tract. Such irritation may be the result of chemical (e.g. alcohol) or microbiological (e.g. *salmonella*); in this respect vomiting can be regarded as an important protective reflex.

- Impulses from the canals in the ear, for instance in motion sickness.

- Brain tumours or a rise in intracranial pressure.

- Higher cerebral centres, as a response to intense anxiety, fear, unpleasant sights or smells.

- Some drugs, for example emetics, such as apomorphine, which can be used in alcohol-aversion therapy.

Vomiting can present the following problems, and so care should be directed towards alleviating the effects these problems pose for patients as well as the cause of vomiting.

- Loss of fluid, and also a loss of those electrolytes present in gastric juice, mainly sodium, chloride and potassium.

- Loss of gastric acid, which can result in a metabolic alkalosis. Similar problems can result from long-term nasogastric drainage, when the gastric aspirate is not replaced.

- Exhaustion and soreness of those muscle groups (described earlier) used in vomiting.

- Weight loss and nutritional disturbances if the vomiting is prolonged.

- A sore throat, as a result of a reflux of acid vomit, together with an unpleasant taste in the mouth.

- Inhalation of vomit. This can be potentially fatal. Nurses should always position unconscious patients in the semi-prone position, so that if they do vomit, the vomitus will drain out of the mouth by gravity and so is less likely to be inhaled into the respiratory tract. Inhalation of vomitus can be a cause of death in the unaccustomed drinker who drinks alcohol heavily (for example, at a party), collapses into an unrousable stupor, vomits without waking and inhales the vomitus.

Useful information can be obtained from an examination of the patient's vomitus. For example if it is faeculent, this may indicate an intestinal obstruction; if altered blood is present, then a peptic ulcer may be suspected; if undigested food is present, then pyloric obstruction may be a problem.

NEUROLOGICAL OBSERVATIONS

The assessment of pain is a complex activity that involves a consideration of physical and psychological aspects of the individual. As outlined in Chapter 3, pain is a subjective experience and the nurse is required to be able to summarise the information provided by the patient against some form of objective criteria. This is essential to evaluate the effectiveness of any pain-relieving interventions. To identify the characteristics of a patient's pain, the nurse should consider the following:

- Type of pain: is it sharp, dull or aching pain?

- Intensity of pain: is it mild, moderate or severe? (Pain assessment scales can be used here.)

- Onset of pain: was it sudden or gradual? What was the patient doing when the pain started?

- Duration of pain: is the pain persistent, constant or intermittent?

- Location of pain: ask patient to be as specific as possible.

- Appearance: is there swelling or discoloration at the pain site?

This provides a very brief summary of some of the issues the nurse should consider when assessing pain.

SUMMARY

A major part of this chapter has been devoted to demonstrating well-established methods by which nurses perform clinical observations. These basic observations are usually taught at fundamental level near the start of training and it is important for student nurses to have a thorough understanding of the significance of these observations. They enable the nurse to make well-informed clinical decisions quickly and accurately. This section has addressed cardiovascular, respiratory, eliminatory and temperature observations. It should be stressed that neurological observations have been omitted from this section, as these are rarely taught in the early part of a nursing curriculum. For information on neurological observations the reader is advised to refer to a more detailed nursing text: Alexander, M. F., Fawcett, J. N. and Runciman, P. J. (2000) *Nursing Practice: Hospital and Home* (Chapter 28 The Unconscious Patient) Edinburgh: Churchill Livingstone.

FURTHER READING

Blows, W. T. (2001) *The Biological Basis of Nursing Clinical Observations*, London: Routledge. See esp. ch. 2.

Grandis, S., Long, G., Glasper, A., and Jackson, P. (2003) *Foundation Studies for Nursing: Using Enquiry-Based Learning*, New York: Palgrave Macmillan.

Hogston, R., and Simpson, P. M. (1999) *Foundations of Nursing Practice*, London: Macmillan Press.

Kenworthy, N., Snowley, G., and Gilling, C. (1992) *Common Foundation Studies in Nursing*, Edinburgh: Churchill Livingstone.

5 SAFETY IN NURSING

The Nursing Midwifery Council (NMC) recently updated the code of professional conduct to provide an unequivocal message to reflect the personal accountability and sense of moral responsibility that nurses must convey in their role. One of the main responsibilities relates to the safety of patients. Many nursing activities carry some risk to the patient, as well as to the nurse. In this chapter several key aspects of safe practice in nursing are addressed. The main emphasis is placed on the safe administration of medication, although control of infection and manual handling are also examined. Safe working practice entails making sure the nurses do not put themselves or their patients at unnecessary risk. One recurrent theme in this chapter is the importance of appropriate hand hygiene. Regardless of levels of experience, from the most junior student to the most senior nurse, hands should ideally be washed after each patient contact. It should be emphasised that each hospital trust will have its own policy to deal with safety issues and students are strongly encouraged to be familiar with these.

DRUG ADMINISTRATION

The administration of drugs by different routes and for various purposes is a common activity in nursing. The guidelines for safe practice are outlined below. When administering drugs, it is important that the nurse ensures that the correct procedures have been followed to protect the patient.

In 2000 the UKCC, now replaced by the NMC, as the nursing professional body produced the *Guidelines for the Administration of Medicines*, which stated that 'in administering any medication, in assisting or overseeing any self administration of medication, you must exercise your professional judgement and apply your knowledge and skill in the given situation'. The statement implies that nurses should have knowledge of the drug they are dispensing, know its effects and potential side effects and assess the suitability for that medication at that given time.

The nursing professional body insists that the administration of medicines should be undertaken by a fully qualified nurse. However, all practitioners, including student nurses, who administer drugs are responsible and accountable for their practice.

Additionally, one of the developing roles in nursing relates to the area of nurse prescription. Prescribing drugs, once the domain of other health professionals, has been introduced and demonstrated to be safe by more senior nurses for selected drugs and preparations to provide more responsive patient care.

In this section, emphasis will be placed upon issues that the student nurse will encounter surrounding the administration of medications.

The five C's of drug administration has been devised for nurses to assist in the safety of this procedure:

- correct patient

- correct drug

- correct dose

- correct time

- correct route.

Correct patient

It is of vital importance for the nurse to check the identity of the patient prior to administration of any drug. All hospital patients wear an identification band, which contains the patient's name, date of birth and a unique hospital number. The details on the identification band should be checked and verified with the patient prior to administration of the drug.

The student is encouraged to consult the *British National Formulary* (BNF) or other pharmaceutical textbooks for more comprehensive information about drugs and their actions.

In hospitals, medicines cannot be administered without a written prescription. Prescriptions should be made by a doctor on a prescription chart and must include:

- the patient's name

- the date the prescription was written

- the medication and the dosage

- the route of administration for the drug

- the time of administration

- specific information about the drug (e.g. whether it should it be taken with meals etc.).

Correct drug

Prescriptions are normally written on a standard prescription sheet, often called the drug kardex. It is the responsibility of the nurse to check the prescription for completeness. The prescription must be legible and signed by the appropriate doctor and the approved generic name of the drug must be used. The difference between generic and trade name can be a source of confusion and nurses may be required to explain to their patients that they are not receiving a new drug. Nurses should also be aware that the names of drugs can be very complex and there are often similarities between names.

With this in mind, it is suggested that medications are checked three times during the administration process:

1. When the drug is taken from the trolley or cabinet.
2. As the drug is matched to the prescription sheet.
3. As the drug is returned to the trolley or cabinet.

To prepare medications for administration it is important that the nurse has clean hands and a clean surface to dispense the drugs from. To prepare the right amount of medication for the patient, the student nurse will have to become familiar with the different Latin abbreviations and measurement systems used in drug administration. It has been suggested that the use of Latin abbreviations be discontinued in clinical practice.

However, they are still commonplace in most clinical areas and include:

p.r.n.	given as necessary	s.c.	subcutaneous
q.i.d.	four times a day	s.l.	sublingual (under tongue)
t.i.d.	three times a day	i.m.	intramuscular
b.d.	twice daily	i.v.	intravenous
p.o.	by mouth	p.r.	by rectum

Controlled drugs are potentially addictive drugs which require closer monitoring and storage in a secure locked cupboard. The nurse in charge of a clinical area carries the keys for this cupboard and holds responsibility for them. Two people are required to be involved in the administration of controlled drugs, one of whom must be a registered nurse. The prescription is checked and administered as for usual medication. Examples of controlled drugs are morphine and pethidine.

Correct time

Most drugs are designed to be given with an interval of several hours apart to provide a consistent therapeutic dose. Therefore, it is essential that drugs are prescribed at regular intervals to maximise the potential of the drug and to avoid unwanted side effects. Drugs are usually given between or just after meals in set drug rounds. To reduce the risk of errors on drug rounds the following structured routine is recommended:

- *Always* use the correct prescription chart.

- *Always* check patient identification thoroughly, even for a well-known patient.

- *Never* administer a drug you did not witness being prepared.

- Do *not* leave a patient's drugs on a locker.

- Do *not* return an unused dose to the original bottle.

- *Never* leave the drug trolley open or unattended.

Increasingly, medications are being stored in locked cupboards at the patient's bedside. Although all the principles of safe drug administration remain, this practice reduces the requirement for drug rounds.

Correct route

All medications are given a specific licence for route of administration. Drugs may be administered in a number of ways, including:

- oral (by mouth)

- rectal (into the rectum)

- topical (on to the skin)

- optic (into the eye)

- nasal (into the nose)

- sublingual (under the tongue)

- vaginal (into the vagina)

- inhalation (via the respiratory tract)

- aural (into the ear)

- intracardiac (into the heart).

Nurses are not responsible for the administration of drugs to all these sites. For example, doctors are involved in the administration of intracardiac drugs.

It is also important to be aware that most drugs are available in more than one form (e.g. tablet, suspension, liquid); the choice of administration is usually based upon rate of absorption required and the patient's general condition.

Calculating drug doses requires the nurse to understand measurement terms. Drugs are measured in grams (g), milligrams (mg) and micrograms (mcg). Measurement of fluid volumes is usually expressed in litres (l) or millilitres (ml).

Oral route
The oral route is the most commonly used route for drug administration. It is the safest, most convenient and least expensive route for medication delivery. Oral medications come in several forms: tablet, capsule, liquids or suspensions (see Figures 4.3 and 4.4). Enteric-coated tablets are covered with a substance that cannot be broken down until the tablet reaches the small intestine. This is to ensure that the active ingredient in the tablet is not released until it is in this region of the body.

The nurse should ensure that the drug trolley is well stocked with specifically prescribed drugs and ensure that these drugs are all well within their expiry dates.

Equipment required on a drug trolley includes:

- medicine pots – to dispense individual medications

- freshly filled water jug – to ensure water is available

- straws – some patients find it easier to swallow

- Drug reference book (*BNF*) – to check unfamiliar doses or drugs.

Guidelines for oral drug administration:

1. Wash hands.
2. Check prescription for date, time, drug to be given and route of drug.
3. Ensure that the nurse has a basic understanding of the effects of drug.
4. Select and check medication, ensuring valid expiry date.
5. Prepare the dosage as prescribed.
6. Re-check labels on container to confirm correct drug has been selected.
7. Take the medication and drug chart to patient.
8. Check patient's identity band and verify with patient.
9. Ensure the patient is positioned upright to aid swallowing.
10. Document the drug dose and time.
11. Dispose of waste and used containers.
12. Monitor patient for efficacy of drug and potential side effects.

Sublingual medication, such as glycerine trinitrate for symptoms of angina, is designed to be released slowly by dissolving under the tongue. The same procedure is followed as with oral medication, but the tablet is placed under the tongue.

Naso-gastric route
Some patients with a naso-gastric (NG) tube have their medication administered through it. The route is suitable for
patients who cannot swallow, but have a functioning gastrointestinal tract. Naso-gastric feeding enables the patient to
take their medication without having to resort to more invasive methods (i.e. injection). Ideally, the medication will be
in liquid form. The drug absorption rate is similar to the oral
route. Drugs should not be added directly to a feed as they may
react with the feed and could potentially block the feeding
tube.

The following procedure should be used when administering drugs via the naso-gastric route:

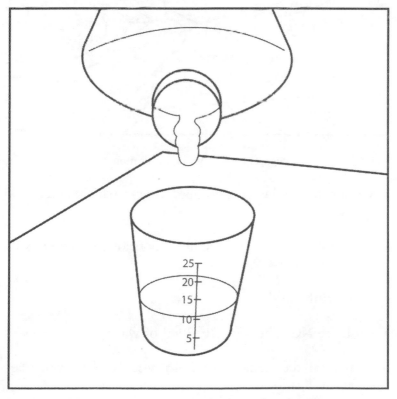

Figure 4.3 Measuring liquid dose of medication

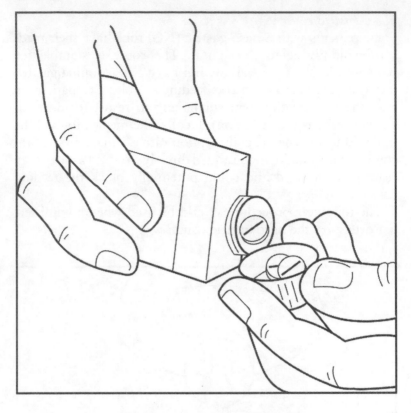

Figure 4.4 Decanting medication

- Wash hands and take prescribed drug to patient and check identity.

- Position patient in a semi-cumbent position to reduce risk of reflux.

- Turn off the feed.

- Flush the NG tube with 20–30ml of water.

- Administer the medication (flush with 10ml of water between medications).

- Reconnect patient to the feeding pump.

Parenteral route
The parenteral route refers to the act of administering drugs by a route other than via the gastrointestinal system. Injection routes such as intramuscular, subcutaneous and intravenous are the most commonly used parenteral routes.

Intramuscular (IM) injections usually deliver medication directly into one of five main sites in the body:

1. deltoid – located in upper arm
2. dorso-gluteal – just above the buttock
3. ventro-gluteal – located in the hip area
4. vastus lateralis – located in thigh muscle
5. rector femoris – located in thigh muscle.

These skeletal muscles are ideal as they are well perfused with blood and have very few pain receptors. The nurse must consider the patient's age prior to the administration of drugs via the intramuscular route: elderly patients may have muscle wasting, which limits the choice of injection site, and babies may have underdeveloped muscles. Therefore the proposed injection site should be checked for:

- sufficient muscle mass

- a good blood supply

- presence of skin damage (potentially from previous injection)

- presence of infection or fibrosis.

There are different syringes and needles (colour-coded) suiting a variety of different procedures. The larger needles are used to reach muscle layers in adults. Gloves should be worn by nurses giving injections to reduce the risk of cross-infection and to avoid contact with drugs.

The student nurse giving an intramuscular injection will require the following equipment:

- a syringe (appropriate size dependent upon amount to be injected)

- two needles (appropriate size for patient and site of injection)

- alcohol swab (if hospital policy)

- gauze swab

- prescribed drug and prescription sheet

- gloves.

Preparation of the injection is an aspectic procedure and requires sterile equipment. The nurse should make every effort to prevent contamination of equipment during procedure. It is important to check that all equipment is sealed and within expiry date.

The drug vial must be checked and prepared. If the drug is stored in a glass ampoule the nurse should use a piece of gauze to break the ampoule to reduce the risk of a glass cut. The next stage involves the assembly of the syringe and the needle; at all stages the nurse must take care to avoid a needle-stick injury. The nurse should always use a clean, dry needle to give the injection. Therefore, any needle that is used to draw up or to dilute the drug should be changed.

It is important that the nurse explains the procedure to the patient to gain his or her co-operation.

The student nurse should then:

- Wash hands and put on gloves.

- Check patient identity.

- Close the curtains to provide privacy.

- Position patient for easy access to injection site.

- If policy dictates, clean skin in location of injection site with alcohol swab.

- Remove the needle cap.

- Position the needle at 90 degrees to skin and insert, using a dart-like action.

- Pull back the plunger of the syringe. If blood is present, withdraw the needle and repeat procedure with a sterile needle.

- If no blood is aspirated, proceed with injection and inject the drug slowly.

- Remove the needle at 90 degrees to skin.

- Apply gentle pressure on the site with alcohol swab.

- Dispose of the needle and syringe as per hospital policy (a dedicated disposal bin, usually a yellow cin bin).

- Do *not* resheaf the needle.

- Discard apron and gloves.

- Complete all necessary prescription records.

There are several complications that can arise from intra-muscular injections. These include risk of infection, muscle damage and nerve damage. It is a nursing responsibility to be aware of the indications of these complications and to make every effort to prevent them.

Subcutaneous injections: very small amounts of medication

can be given into subcutaneous (below the skin) tissue to allow a slow, sustained absorption of medications. One group of patients who use this route to inject insulin are diabetics. The main sites for administering subcutaneous injections include the upper arm, the abdomen, the outer area of the thigh and the back (see Figure 4.5). Nurses can also use inject subcutaneously on the upper buttocks and outer thighs but these areas are not accessible for patients to self-administer.

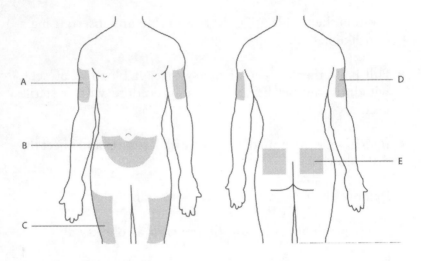

Figure 4.5 Injection sites (subcutaneous)

The student nurse giving a subcutaneous injection will require the following equipment:

● a syringe (insulin or 1ml syringe)

● two needles (appropriate size for patient and site of injection)

● alcohol swab (if hospital policy)

● gauze swab

- prescribed drug and prescription sheet

- gloves.

It is important that the nurse explains the procedure to the patient to gain his or her co-operation.
The student nurse should then:

- Wash hands and put on gloves.

- Check patient identity.

- Close the curtains to provide privacy.

- Position patient for easy access to injection site.

- If policy dictates, clean skin in location of injection site with alcohol swab.

- Remove needle cap.

- Grasp the skin between the thumb and forefinger and pinch a fold of fatty tissue away from muscle.

- Insert needle at 45 or 90 degrees depending upon size of needle used.

- Release skin fold and inject slowly and steadily.

- Dispose of the needle and syringe as per hospital policy (yellow cin bin).

- Discard apron and gloves.

- Complete all necessary prescription records.

Topical medication

Topical administration of medication refers to the application of substances to the skin or mucous membranes to achieve local or systemic effects. Topical medications are available in several formats such as an oil, lotion or cream.

Rectal medication

The rectal route of administration of medication is frequently used in adults and children. Rectal administration of medication by-passes the upper gastrointestinal tract. This avoids the need to metabolise the drug in the liver and therefore ensures that the drug will act more quickly. Rectal medications come in the form of suppository, cream or solution and are usually prescribed for patients who are unable to swallow or who are unconscious. Enemas and suppositories to relieve constipation are examples of drugs given via the rectal route.

Vaginal medication

Vaginal medications come in several forms: pessaries, creams and douches. These usually can only be administered with special applicators.

Opthalmic medication

Opthalmic medication relates to the administration of drugs into the eyes. Eye medications usually come in two forms: eye drops or ointments. These may be used to treat specific eye conditions (e.g. glaucoma) or to aid in the diagnosis of eye conditions. The administration of eye medication in hospital is often the responsibility of the nurse, who will also be responsible for teaching the patient or relatives how to administer the medication. The following guidelines outline the principles for administration of eye medications:

- To prevent cross-infection, separate containers should be used for each eye.

- If eye drops and ointment are prescribed to be administered at the same time, the nurse should be given the drops first, followed by ointment ten minutes later. Ointment may prevent the absorption of eye drops.

- Medication should *not* be directed on to the cornea of the eye; this may cause damage.

- If the nurse is clearing discharge from the eye, dry cotton wool should not be used, as fibres may get into the eye and cause further discomfort.

- The nurse should *always* work from the nose side outwards when applying ointment or swabbing the eye, to reduce risk of infection.

- If both eyes have to be treated but only one is infected, treat the cleaner eye first to prevent cross-infection. Wash hands between treating each eye.

The student nurse administering eye medication will require the following equipment:

- prescribed drug and prescription sheet

- gauze swabs

- sterile saline solution and sterile eye-dressing pack

- gloves.

It is important that the nurse explains the procedure to the patient to gain his or her co-operation.

The student nurse should then:

- Follow standard procedure for drug administration.

- Wash hands and put on gloves.

- Check patient identity.

- Position patient (ideally lying flat with head tilted backwards).

- Check the eye and clean as required.

- Gently pull down the lower eyelid to form a pouch. Insert the number of drops prescribed into the pouch.

- Ask patient to close eye gently and to blink several times.

- The patient should be advised not to rub eyes.

- Remove gloves and wash hands.

- Complete all necessary prescription records.

PATIENT COMPLIANCE

Nurses should be aware that drug therapy can only be effective if the patient co-operates or complies. Failure to complete a course of medication, or comply with treatment, may result in a poor outcome for the patient. There are several steps nurses can take to ensure that patients comply with their treatment regime:

- Good patient education (why it is important to take the medication).

- Provide a written record of drug regime.

- Commence self-administration while in the hospital.

- Involve relatives in the education process.

INFECTION CONTROL

Hospital-acquired infections, known as nosocomial infections, are the source of a great deal of concern because of the associated significant morbidity and mortality.

With an increasingly elderly population, who have a greater susceptibility to infections, nurses have a role to play in the control of infection. As people get older they produce fewer white blood cells, which increase their susceptibility to infection.

The most common type of nosocomial infections are:

- urinary tract (often related to catheterised patients)

- lower respiratory tract

- skin and wounds.

These infections include MRSA (Methicillin-Resistant Staphy (ococcus aureus), *E. Coli* and *salmonella*. As the largest element of the workforce in the National Health Service, with the closest direct contact with patients, nurses are in a unique position to integrate infection control strategies into their nursing practice. It is believed that up to 30 per cent of hospital-based infections could be avoided with the implementation of basic measures to reduce the risk of acquiring infections while in hospital care. As the most likely source of transmission of infectious organisms from body fluid is by direct contact, these basic nursing measures should include:

- Good hand hygiene.

- Disposable gloves to be worn when dealing with all patient's body fluids.

- Avoiding direct contact with wounds and dressings.

- Following hospital infection control policy (e.g. catheter care).

- Ensuring hospital equipment for use on patients is sterile or disinfected.

- Disposing of hospital waste and linen as per protocol.

- Maintaining general standards of cleanliness.

As it is impossible to know which patients are infected, it is suggested that the following measures, devised by the Department of Health, should be viewed as universal precautions embodying the principles of good nursing practice in the control and spread of infection:

- Skin – cuts or abrasions should be covered with waterproof dressing.

- Gloves – wear gloves if in contact with body fluids (e.g. blood, urine, saliva, vomit, faeces).

- Hand-washing – thorough hand-washing between all procedures is essential (see below).

- Aprons – should be worn if there is a possibility of splashing.

- Eyes – eye protection should be worn if there is a high risk of splashing. If eyes are splashed, irrigate with water.

- Needle-stick – follow guidelines to avoid accidental injury.

- Spillages – follow local guidelines to deal with spillages.

- Waste – all waste products should be disposed of according to hospital policy.

Most hospital-acquired infections are spread by contact: the hands are a major vehicle in the transmission of infection. Normal skin has a resident population of micro-organisms, and through nursing care with patients, these micro-organisms can be picked up and shed during contact. The main aim of hand-washing in nursing is to remove these transient micro-organisms below the level of an infected dose before they can be transmitted to a patient. The Royal College of Nursing recommends the following guidelines with regard to hand-washing:

- Wash thoroughly with antiseptic detergent (or a 70 per cent alcohol rub).

- Dry with soft, high quality disposable tissues.

- Removal of jewellery prior to hand-washing.

- Nails should be kept short and clean.

Indications for nurses to wash their hands include:

- after handling body fluids

- before and after any invasive procedures

- after handling contaminated items (e.g. bed linen)

- prior to the administration of drugs

- before contact with susceptible patients (e.g. those with low resistance)

- prior to contact with food

- at the beginning and end of every shift.

Soiled and contaminated hospital linen can be a major source of infection in hospitals. Therefore the nurse is responsible for bagging linen at source when removed from the patient's bed and to dispose of the linen in line with hospital policy.

Within the hospital environment, domestic and clinical waste is likely to support the growth of potentially harmful bacteria. Waste products are generally classified according to the following categories:

- domestic waste

- clinical waste (e.g. dressings and swabs)

- sharps (all needles and sharp instruments)

- human tissue requiring incineration.

It is also a nursing responsibility to ensure that patient's hands are kept clean. The nurse should offer the patient hand-washing facilities after visiting the toilet, before meals and at any other time that it is requested.

FOOD HYGIENE

The nurse plays a multiplicity of roles to ensure that the patients are fed safely. In the ward environment this may include food preparation, food handling and assisting patients to eat their meals. Any breaches in hygiene can result in food poisoning.

In recent years there has been a significant rise in certain types of food poisoning, such as *Escherichia coli* (*E. Coli*) and *salmonella typhimurium*. These are examples of multi-resistant bacteria and are difficult to treat with common antibiotics. A variety of diseases can be caused by ingesting food which is contaminated with pathogenic bacteria. Diarrhoea, vomiting and abdominal pain are the most common symptoms of food poisoning. Nurses have responsibility to ensure that patients are appropriately and safely fed. This role involves:

- Meals being served immediately when they arrive in a clinical area.

- Keeping the temperature of hot food above 63°C.

- Ensuring that microwaves are *never* used to reheat or cook food.

- Cold food being kept cold below 5°C.

Nurses with a good knowledge of the sources of food-poisoning bacteria and the most common routes of contamination can take appropriate precautions to reduce the risk of infection. This involves appropriate hand-washing:

- before touching food

- after using the toilet

- after handling waste and bed pans

- covering cuts and sores.

Additionally, equipment and eating utensils should be kept as clean as possible and nurses should try to touch food as little as possible.

MANUAL HANDLING

Manual handling relates to the role of the nurse in the moving of patients. For a student nurse preparing to start a professional career, it is important to be aware of the principles of manual handling guidelines. The safety of the nurse and patient is of vital importance and nurses are educated on handling operations and given guidance on local practice and the use of handling equipment. When moving patients, the aim is to actively encourage independent movement, the nurse assisting as little as possible. Any normal movement that the patients can undertake for themselves avoids the need for lifting, and patient preferences should be taken into account. Due to the risk of injury, the Royal College of Nursing (1995) recommended that nurses in the hospital or community environment should no longer have to lift manually. There is now a wide range of specialised equipment that aids manual handling, for example patient-lifting slings, hard blocks, roller towels and transfer slides. Such equipment minimises the risk of injury.

It is not the intention of this text to fully examine the principles of patient handling and, as these may vary from one hospital to another, readers are encouraged to refer to their local manual handling policy.

SUMMARY

In this chapter some of the key aspects of safe practice in nursing have been examined. From safety in the administration of drugs through to preventing cross infection, it is clear that many nursing procedures carry considerable risk. It is hoped that by following the principles described in this chapter the student nurse can ensure that nursing procedures are carried out safely.

PART II
Study Skills

6 BE IN THE KNOW

INTRODUCTION

Whether you enter university directly from school or as a mature student you may be apprehensive about adapting to a different way of studying at university. It is hoped that the following chapter will provide many helpful hints to help you cope with the rigours of university life.

You cannot settle down to study effectively unless you know what you are doing and why you are doing it. At all levels – what you are doing with your life, what you are doing at university, what you are doing in a hospital ward or in a community health centre – the more informed and aware you are, the better will be your motivation and your ability to study. This introduction aims to take some of the worry out of daily life. Do not be surprised to find, among the information on study skills, a number of hints on what might be described as life skills. For the time you are at university, the two are inextricably linked.

BE IN THE KNOW ABOUT YOUR SUBJECT

The course booklet

Most courses have a course booklet with essential information such as course content, reading lists, a timetable, what the assessment procedures are, whether or not you have to register for exams and, if so, where and when. The course booklet may also tell you how essays and other written work should be presented and outline the style of referencing that is required. Always read the class booklet carefully, and refer to it from time to time, just to remind yourself of what you should be doing at any given point in the term.

The noticeboard

Find out where the class noticeboard is and keep a regular eye on it. Any changes to class times and locations will be posted there, sometimes at short notice. It is the place to look for tutorial lists, exam details and so on. In nursing departments the noticeboard may also contain important information about clinical placements or visits.

The departmental secretary

The departmental office may not be open to student enquiries all day. Find out when the secretary is available. This is where to go if you miss a lecture and need the handout, if you want to double-check dates and places for exams, if you can't get hold of a particular lecturer or if you change your address and so on.

Computing support

Even if you are a complete technophobe, you must find out how to make the most of the available computing facilities. Increasingly, university departments insist that written work be done on a word processor. Some even ask for work to be submitted in an electronic form so that it may be scanned for plagiarism.

On a more positive note, a word processor makes editing and revising your work very much easier; you have the benefit of a spell checker; and you produce an attractive final copy, which will put the marker in a good mood. For larger pieces of work, such as dissertations and theses, the word processor may provide an appropriate layout.

There will almost certainly be courses on computing for new

students and they are well worth going to, whether you are computer literate or a complete beginner. You will save a lot of time and effort if you find out how much your computer can do for you. The infinitely patient, computing-support personnel are equally good at helping nervous beginners and more adventurous, technically minded users.

The computer is also essential for gathering information from library catalogues and from the internet.

You will probably be given an e-mail address in your first week. Check your e-mail frequently because this is how your tutors, lecturers or the departmental secretary will get in touch if they need to contact you urgently, and it will be appreciated by your tutor if you send an e-mail if you have to miss a class.

Before you even apply to a university, explore the websites of universities you might consider going to. They might help you decide which university to chose.

You may also wish to access information about the teaching hospital that is attached to the university that you have an interest in. It is more than likely that you will spend a great deal of your clinical placement in that setting.

7 LEARNING

READING

Your lecturers will recommend reading to be done along with the lecture course. You will get the most out of the lectures and the reading if they keep pace with each other. Sometimes, a lecture course will follow a set textbook quite closely but there will almost certainly be additional reading so that you can broaden your knowledge of the subject and assess different points of view.

Your first task is to get hold of the book or article. There will be some texts that are recommended for purchase and, knowing that students are always short of money, lecturers will keep this list to a minimum. Watch the noticeboards for second-hand copies. If you are tempted to buy an old edition, check with your tutor that there have not been too many changes. Books that you do not have to buy will be in the library. Make sure that you are first in the queue. There are always more students than books. Right from the start, get to know your library and how it works. Get to know the shelf numbers where nursing and health books are kept. Practise using the online catalogue. It will tell you not only where to find books, but also whether they have been borrowed and when they are due back. If a book that you need has been borrowed, you may be able to recall it. Just ask at the service desk. There may be more than one place to find books. For example, there are the ordinary open shelves (or stacks) that make up most of the library, but, in addition, especially when books are recommended for essays and there is likely to be a huge demand for them, books may be put in a special section of the library where they are on very short loans, say three hours at a time. Many large hospitals have good library resources and this can often be a useful source of material for student nurses. If you have problems, the most valuable resource in a library is the librarian. Ask a member of the library staff for help.

The best academic writers, particularly those who are directing their writing towards first-year students, try very hard to keep their writing clear and easy to read. However, it is not always possible to express very complex ideas in very simple language. Furthermore, learning a new subject means learning all the terminology of that subject. Occasionally, some of the reading that you do will be very dry and difficult. Persist. Gradually, you will build up your reading muscles to Olympic standards. This is yet another of the benefits of a university education; no Act of parliament, company report or small print on a contract will daunt you after graduation.

The first part of this book will have given you some indication of the type of reading you will have to do, ranging from social to biological science. From it you can see that some topics are more readable that others, but none of it is exactly bedtime-story stuff. It demands what is called 'active reading'. You really have to work and think along with the text. For this reason, do not underestimate how long a chapter will take and do not set yourself too big a chunk of reading in one sitting. Apart from the introductory chapter of each book, you are unlikely to be able to read a chapter straight through from beginning to end. Take a bit at a time. If there are exercises in the book you are reading, do the exercises for each section as you go along. If there are no exercises, set yourself some. Take notes. Try to rephrase the text in your own words as you do so. Occasionally, joint study sessions with other members of your tutorial group might be helpful. Together, you might make more sense of difficult passages, come up with good examples, or be able to test each other.

The moment you sit down with a book, make sure you note down all the necessary bibliographical detail (see 'Further Reading' sections in this book for examples), including page numbers. Be sure to mark exact quotations in your notes. If you find something you may wish to quote word for word, make sure that you get every detail right, including the punctuation. If it contains what looks like an error, put 'sic' after the error and then everyone will know that you are quoting accurately and the mistake is not yours. Much of your note-taking will consist of paraphrases or summaries of the text but often a passage from a book will spark off your own ideas. Make a note of the passage and write down your responses to the passage at once, or you will almost certainly forget what they were. Be sure that you make it very clear which notes are exact quotes, which are paraphrases and which are your own thoughts. (Use different colours of pen.) It is very easy, at a later date, to think an idea is your own when, in fact, you have picked it up in the course of your reading. Strangely, it is even possible to have an original idea and then to convince yourself that you read it somewhere.

Notes are an aid to learning, not a substitute for it. You should not just copy down words for future reference. Try to take notes in your own words. Before you can do that, you have to understand what you have read, and this is the first step in learning. The physical act of writing something down will help to fix it in your mind. Also, you have to be selective and, in being selective, you begin to exercise your critical judgement. If you then take notes of your notes, you repeat these learning steps. If you are using your own book or a photocopy, you will probably use highlighter pen. Do not be tempted to use highlighter or underlining as a way of not having to read something that you suspect is important but is too hard to understand. Make the effort then and there. If it is important enough to highlight, it is important enough to learn. Do not highlight indiscriminately or you will not be able to see the wood for the trees.

Only once you have done the recommended reading should you start looking for additional reading. The set books might make recommendations, or you could browse along the library shelves, or you could do a search on the library online catalogue. Subject searches are not always reliable. Sometimes keywords in the title can produce better results. This might produce such a wealth of material that you don't know where to start. A good guide is the number of times a book or article is cited in other people's bibliographies. You will see from this which texts are important reading. If you need help, ask your tutor.

When you are browsing, use the contents page or abstract to identify useful and interesting bits and scan-read to find the bits you want. Do not start at the beginning and try to work your way through. First make sure that the book or article has something to offer.

Get to know the major works of reference, such as the *Oxford English Dictionary*, or K. Wilkie and I. Burns (2003) *Problem-Based Learning: A Handbook for Nurses*, London: Palgrave Macmillan.

If you want to photocopy anything, you must obey the regulations on copyright displayed beside university photocopying machines.

LEARNING BY ASSESSMENT

There are two kinds of assessment, formative and summative. The formative assessment counts towards your final mark but it also, even more importantly, provides you with the feedback you need to improve your performance and get the most out of the course. The summative assessment is the final test of what you have learned during the course.

The most usual ways of assessing student performance in nursing are essays, exercises and examinations. There may be a small proportion of marks for tutorial participation. Most institutions now use continuous assessment, which means that classwork counts towards the final mark. In some departments, you may even be granted exemption from the degree examination if your coursework is of a very high standard.

Exams and essays usually give a very generous amount of choice. This practice can leave a large part of the course unexamined in any way. Therefore, some course organisers prefer to set assignments which require short answers to questions covering a much greater proportion of the course curriculum. These assignments are not necessarily set under exam conditions but might take the place of a class exam. All the comments in Chapters 12 and 13 apply equally well to assignments.

Whatever form your assessed classwork takes, the marks are for your benefit as much as for the examiners' benefit. The class booklet should tell you what the marks really mean in terms of whether you have just passed, or passed well, or passed outstandingly. Go by what the class booklet says rather than by comparing yourself with other students. Some years seem to produce a larger number of good students than other years, but the marking criteria stay the same. Look at the markers' comments, good as well as bad, and try to see what makes a good nursing answer. If a few of you can get together and go over marked essays, exams or assignments, you will get a better picture of what markers are looking for.

PROBLEM-BASED LEARNING

Many nursing institutions have adopted problem-based learning (PBL) in various forms to establish more student-centred and humanistic approaches to nurse education.

Problem-based learning is an increasingly popular method of education, commonly used at undergraduate level. PBL is a very general term that is used to describe an approach to learning in which students working in small groups facilitated by tutors identify their own learning objectives from scenarios. It is a combination of educational method and philosophy, which encourages nurse tutors to rethink and change their educational role away from one in which they predominantly convey facts. PBL aims to enable students to acquire and structure knowledge in an efficient, accessible and integrated way. It is clear that such methods are not apparent through traditional forms of teaching where the student plays a more passive role.

However in the case of PBL student activity is encouraged. Scenario-based learning includes several elements of PBL:

- Learning and teaching come from an exposure to a scenario.

- Small interactive groups of students explore the scenario in a structured manner and subsequently share the knowledge and understanding.

- A non-didactic facilitator.

Although not utilised in all educational institutions, PBL is a common feature in many nursing courses in universities.

SELF-DIRECTED LEARNING

Libraries are usually good places to work, if you can manage to ignore occasional, irritating whisperers. You are less likely to fidget and go off to do other things than you are at home. You are not going to be distracted by flatmates, visits to the fridge or your favourite television programme. If you are used to working in the library, you get into the habit of using it in breaks between classes, potentially useful time which can easily be frittered away.

If you live with other students, make sure that there are clear rules about not interrupting each other's study time. People who play very loud music at three in the morning before a flatmate's exam are not appreciated. Be considerate about your flatmates' exams and essay deadlines and make sure they do the same for you.

By now you will be aware of the length of time that you can work without a break. You are unlikely to be working effectively if you go for much more than an hour without a rest. You can keep your concentration up for longer if you vary your tasks. Read and note-take for a bit. Then do some practical exercises or test yourself in some other way before going back to reading again. Remember not to set yourself too much reading in one go.

Sit down to study with a realistic target in mind. Reward yourself (with a rest, a shower, a computer game, a chat with friends or a phonecall) when you have achieved your goal.

Try to avoid working late at night. If you find that it is becoming a habit, revise your time management. If you do find yourself burning the midnight oil, and all students do from time to time, strong black coffee or other highly caffeinated drinks are not the answer. They may give you a short boost, but they will leave you even more tired and so you have another cup, and another. The result is that when you finally go to bed, you can't sleep and you will probably get a headache as well. Try herbal tea or a few deep breaths at an open window instead.

8 TIME MANAGEMENT

Time management is one of the transferable skills that employers value in a university graduate.

As you progressed through school, you will gradually have been given more and more responsibility for your own time management, but, between school and university, there is a great chasm. You were expected to get to school at the same time every morning and stay there and work until everybody went home. If you were not at a class, somebody wanted to know where you were. Homework was given in comparatively small regular amounts and woe betide you if it was not done.

At university, you may not have a class every day. You may start at nine in the morning, but you might not start until the afternoon. The strict routine of school disappears. You have to make sure you establish a good new routine. Bad time managers start getting up late, missing classes, working late to try to meet deadlines and end up feeling permanently tired, miserable and inadequate. Time management starts when the alarm clock goes off. You need to establish a daily routine.

You also need to keep an eye on the bigger time-management picture. If you were a course organiser, how would you work out the deadline for handing in essays? You can't set an essay too early in the course because the work has not been covered. You want to hand marked essays back in time for students to learn from them before the exams. All course organisers think this way and so the deadlines for essays for all your subjects have a nasty habit of falling around the same time. It is no excuse to say, 'I had three essays to hand in for today. I haven't finished my Human Biology one. Please can I have an extension?' The time between the setting of the essay and the deadline is very generous, perhaps as much as five weeks. The time to get started is as soon as possible after the essay topics are given out. Furthermore, being quick off the mark means that you get to the library before all the books on the reading list disappear.

Some subjects you can swot up the week before exams and use flair or common sense to fill in the gaps. Nursing is not one of them. It is not a difficult subject but it involves skills which have to be practised and built up over a period of time. If you keep up with lectures and tutorials and do the exercises that are set, you will find the exams are really not a problem.

You can improve your exam technique greatly by planning how much time you are going to spend on each question and sticking to it. You know the duration of the exam and you know the number of questions. Assuming that each question is worth the same number of marks, you simply divide the time equally among the questions. This may sound obvious, but it is amazing how many students make a mess of exams because they don't do it.

As you write an exam answer, you pick up marks very rapidly in the first ten or fifteen minutes of writing. After that, the rate at which you collect marks slows down and eventually you reach a plateau. There may even come a point when you end up exposing your ignorance instead of showing off your knowledge and your marks could begin to drop. So, obviously, it is better to start three questions than to finish two and leave one unstarted. Before you start practising for exams, work out how much time you can have for each question. Remember to allow for the time it takes to put your name on the paper and to fill in the other administrative details, question-reading time, thinking time and essay-plan time. For essay-type answers, note the time at which you must start to draw each question to a close. Even if you have not completely finished when your time is up, move ruthlessly on to the next question. You may have time to go back and finish it later. Usually, each answer is written in a separate book, but, if this is not the case, leave a big space between answers so that you can go back and add any necessary finishing touches. If there are questions which are divided into sections, work out how much time you can afford to spend on each section and pace yourself accordingly. If you have practised on past papers, you may find that there are some questions you can do quite quickly. When it comes to the exam, do the quick ones first and divide up the time you have saved among the remaining questions.

If you have had to get a job in order to pay your way through university, keep your priorities clear. University comes first. When you start missing classes to go to work, something has gone wrong.

Finally, remember to plan some time for relaxation. If you deliberately leave time for having a bit of fun, then you will not be so tempted to let your relaxation time eat into your working time.

9 TUTORIALS, SEMINARS AND ORAL PRESENTATIONS

TUTORIALS

Tutorials are probably the most efficient and enjoyable way of learning. They usually consist of a small group of students and a tutor. Right from the beginning, get to know at least some of the people in your tutorial group. It can be a great help to go for coffee after a tutorial and talk about nursing and health care with people who are at the same stage as you. It means that you will have people you know to sit next to in lectures. It also means that, if for any reason you have to miss a lecture, you can borrow lecture notes easily.

The official aims of a tutorial are to reinforce lectures, to clarify any points in the lectures that you did not understand and to explore topics in more depth than can be attempted in lectures, perhaps moving on to related topics that were not covered in the lecture but which are still relevant to the course. To get the most out of a tutorial, you need to tell your tutor where your difficulties and interests lie.

Do not be afraid of asking something silly or giving a wrong answer. In tutorials, you are very unlikely be assessed on what you know (although you should clarify any criteria for assessment with your tutor). If tutors award a mark for tutorial performance at all (and not all courses have tutorial assessment) it will be based on attendance and participation. If you make a mistake in a tutorial, you and your tutor can get to the bottom of it and clear up any misunderstandings. Better to make a mistake there than in the exams or essays.

Attendance at tutorials is usually compulsory and if your attendance is poor, the tutor will be obliged to inform the course organiser and your director of studies or personal tutor. This is partly for academic reasons, to make sure you are not falling behind with your work. It is also for pastoral reasons, to make sure you not ill or in some kind of difficulty. Please try to let your tutor know if you are going to be absent. Believe it or not, your tutor will worry about you. Because tutors are the members of university staff that students come into contact with most frequently, they are often the first person that a student will consult about a non-academic problem.

Discussion plays a large part in tutorials. Each tutor has his or her own style of teaching, but you may well find that you spend a lot of time in your first year practising the skills required to write a clinical diary. Your problem-solving skills will undoubtedly be extended.

Your tutor may well give you some clues about essay writing. If your tutor spends part of a tutorial giving a taught lesson rather than a discussion or practical session, look for structure. Can you spot possible section headings for an essay? If you are stuck with your essay, seek help from your tutor. Do not expect any help that would give you an unfair advantage, but your tutor may be able to discuss the topic with you in a very general way and sometimes the very act of explaining your difficulty to someone who understands can make you solve your problem yourself.

In the last tutorial before the exams, keep your ears tuned in for clues. Your tutor may be authorised to tell you a bit about the exam layout. You may go over old papers in the tutorial and be given hints on question spotting or hints on structuring answers. If the course has changed recently, past papers can put you in a complete panic by asking about things you have not covered, and your tutor will be able to reassure you. If the tutor does some exam revision with you, which topics are the focus of attention? After the exam, be sure to ask your tutor about any mistakes you have made if you cannot see for yourself how to put them right.

The better prepared you are for a tutorial, the more you will get out of it. Obviously, you will do any reading that the tutor has asked you to do and you should attempt any exercises that you are given as homework. It is not unusual for students to find some exercises very difficult at first. If that happens, do as

much as you can and try to work out exactly where you are
getting stuck. Let your tutor see your attempt, however
pathetic it looks to you. Do not be embarrassed. You are
not going to be the only one in the group who gets stuck. The
tutor needs to know what areas of the course require extra
consolidation and which bits are easy enough for you to revise
on your own. If there is no set homework, make sure that you
have understood the lectures and the recommended reading
that goes with them. Tell the tutor about the bits that are not
clear.

If you have any special needs, tell your tutors if there is
anything they can do to help. For example, if you are partially
deaf and need to lip read, suggest to the tutor that you sit
where you can see the tutor's face clearly, in good lighting, and
ask the tutor to help by speaking clearly. If the tutor lapses and
starts talking to the blackboard, a quick reminder will not
cause any offence and would actually be appreciated by the
tutor.

SEMINARS

Between the full-scale large lecture and the small, intimate
tutorial lies the seminar. It is a rather vague term because
different teachers approach seminars in different ways. Some
treat them as large tutorials and others treat them as small
lectures. There should be more opportunity for questions and
comments in a seminar, so come well prepared in order to
contribute but, because it is a larger gathering, you must also
let other people speak and take care not to monopolise the
teacher's time. Do not expect the same level of individual
attention that you get in tutorials.

ORAL PRESENTATIONS

Some tutors expect students to give oral presentations in
tutorials. It is not very likely that this will happen at the start

of first year. By the time you have to give a talk, you will be familiar with your subject and friendly with the other members of the tutorial group, who are all going to have to go through the same torment.

Your oral presentation will be based on a written paper, produced with all the skills you would use for writing an essay. Many tutors will be quite content if you simply read from your written paper. Your fellow students, on the other hand, will be bored to tears. So:

- Try to keep your voice interested and interesting.

- Be sufficiently well prepared so that your nose is not always buried in your paper.

- Mark the important points in your paper (probably topic sentences) with a highlighter pen, so that you can find your way at a glance.

- As you speak, watch your fellow students and make eye contact with them and the tutor.

- Smile.

- Invite questions and comments and be prepared to deal with them.

- Do not be afraid to admit that you do not have all the answers.

- With your tutor's permission, make use of any appropriate audio-visual aids (whiteboard, overhead projector, computer screen, recordings).

- Provide a handout if you think it would be useful.

10 LECTURES

First-year nursing classes can be quite large. A certain amount of noise is inevitable, particularly during the winter term when everybody seems to have coughs and colds. Coughs, inexplicably, get worse during lectures. Therefore, it is a good idea to arrive in good time and get a seat quite near the front where there is less chance of being distracted and you will be able to hear. If the lecturer is inaudible or if the visual aids are not visible, let the lecturer know at once. If you have a hearing problem consult the university's special-needs advisor. If you have a motor or visual problem and cannot take notes, ask the lecturer if you can use a tape-recorder. Tape-recorders should not be used by anyone without permission.

Lecturing styles vary quite a lot and so you must be able to adapt your note-taking and listening. Most lecturers provide a course outline in the class booklet and it is a good idea to take a look at this and get a general picture of where the lecturers are heading. Some lecturers follow a published book (sometimes their own). If there is not a suitable book to refer to, you may well get a handout at the lecture or handouts may be collected in a class booklet. If there is such a class booklet make sure you take it with you. If the lecturer sticks closely to the handout, it might be enough just to make marginal notes on it. If there is no handout, or if the handout is extra to the content of the lecture, be sure to take notes. You may think you will remember it all but you won't. A good lecturer will have planned the lecture and it will have a structure. In fact, even although the lecturer may sound quite spontaneous, the lecture should have been constructed in sections and paragraphs like a well-thought-out essay. The lecturer may tell you the gameplan at the start of the lecture. Try to structure your notes accordingly. Use bullet points and numbers where possible. Use a different coloured pen to highlight key terms and VIPs (Very Important Points). This will help with exam revision. You would be very exceptional if your concentration did not lapse occasionally in lectures, but train yourself to waken up rapidly if the lecturer gives any VIP signals.

Not all lecturers are charismatic and riveting. You may have to make a big effort to stop your attention from wandering. On these occasions, you could try active rather than passive listening. Imagine you are in a radio discussion programme and you are going to have to respond to what the lecturer is saying. What can you agree with? What would you question? What stimulates you to think in fresh directions? Not only will this game help to keep you awake but it will also help you to take good notes.

At the end of a lecture, there will probably be a short time for questions. Do not be afraid to ask. If, however, you cannot bring yourself to speak in front of a large audience, have a private word with the lecturer afterwards. Questions are useful feedback for lecturers, who need to know whether their lectures are pitched at the right level.

Always take a look over, and make sense of, your lecture notes the same night, while the lecture is still fresh in your mind and, if there is recommended reading to do, do it as soon as possible after the lecture. You might like to revise your lecture notes with a friend, in the hope that your absent moments do not coincide and that, if one of you has a gap in your notes, the other can supply the deficiency. By the same token, if you miss a lecture, borrow notes for the same lecture from at least two people.

Make a special effort to get to the last lecture of every lecture block or module. This is when you might pick up hints about exam questions.

11 ESSAYS AND DISSERTATIONS

You did not get as far as considering university entrance without having gained some skill in writing, but learning to write well is a lifelong task. During your time at university, you will be expected to polish your formal writing style and adapt to the particular conventions of the subject you are writing about.

At university, you will be assessed primarily on what you write and that is inseparable from how you write, because it does not matter how much you know if you cannot get that knowledge down on paper in a way that makes sense to the reader.

Make the most of available technology. Many university departments insist on the use of word processors for essays and you should take advantage of computing courses for new students.

WHY WRITE ESSAYS?

The obvious answer is 'to prove that you have learnt something'. That, however, is not the only or the best answer. If you tackle your essays in the right way, you will find that they are, in fact, a very important part of the learning process. It is only when you try to explain things in a totally clear and unambiguous way that you begin to expose little gaps in your understanding. So you have to go off and consolidate your learning. More encouragingly, you may find that, as you arrange your ideas, you make connections that you had not seen before. You are putting what you have learnt to work and gaining confidence in handling your new knowledge. The more effort you put into an essay, the more you will benefit.

Essay writing at university level demands knowledge of the conventions of academic discourse and especially of the way of writing accepted within the academic circle of your particular subject. All academic discourse demands attention to detail, not just in the facts and theories you present but also in the manner of presentation. A consistent level of formality is required and an impersonal style where the writer does not get in the way of the subject. Vocabulary and grammar have to be carefully checked to make sure there is no possibility of misunderstandings. Bibliographies and sources have to be cited. You are handling complicated ideas and having to express them clearly. In short, you are becoming expert in the transferable skills of gathering, selecting, organising and communicating information.

Essay writing is a very important part of the learning process.

FIRST READ THE QUESTION

More good students get bad marks because they have misread the question than for any other reason. There are certain recognisable types: *Discuss* . . . *Compare and contrast* . . . *Describe* . . . *Analyse* . . . etc. Think about it. Make sure you undertake the activity asked for.

Everything you write must be relevant to the question. If you include irrelevancies, they will not gain marks and they will even lose marks by taking up space that should have been used on answering the question. Word limits on essays are based on the assumption that every word is necessary and to the point. Lecturers think very, very hard about the exact wording of questions. If you are in any doubt what an essay question means, do not be afraid to ask whoever set it.

Chose your question wisely. With experience, you will discover the kind of question you are best at.

THE WRITING PROCESS

Writing is not a single big task. It is a lot of little tasks:

- collecting data

- finding a structure

- making a draft

- polishing

- preparing for submission

- proof-reading.

COLLECTING DATA

Sources

Most of the information you need will have been covered in lectures and reinforced in tutorials. A good essay, however, shows signs of additional reading which has obviously been well understood and used appropriately.

Make sure you can use libraries to the best advantage. Find your way around online catalogues. If you can't find what you are looking for, or don't even know where to start looking, ask the librarians. They will be happy to tell you what is available. You can surf the net for sources including databases which are available to higher education institutions within the UK, such as MEDLINE, etc. For a list of internet sources, see Winship and McNab (1998). A word of warning: especially in the early stages, you can be overwhelmed with sources of information and you may not yet know enough to be selective. This is why your teachers provide recommended reading lists. Use them.

Taking notes for essays

When taking notes, keep the exact wording of the essay title in front of you. Constantly ask yourself, 'How does what I'm reading relate to the title?' Noting down your initial reactions to what you are reading can be a good way of getting into the actual writing of your essay.

Since academic writing demands that you provide proper bibliographies listing all the works you have consulted, it is particularly important that you record all the necessary bibliographic details. If you take something off the internet, make sure you record the website and the date you accessed it.

Only if you are using your own photocopies are highlighter pens acceptable! Remember not to break copyright rules when you are photocopying. The rules should be clearly displayed near the university photocopiers. If in doubt, ask a librarian.

FINDING A STRUCTURE

Students are usually surprised at how much importance markers attach to the structure of essays. Anybody can regurgitate facts. That is not what essay writing is about. Markers are looking for the ability to put the facts to work. Different subjects place a slightly different emphasis on the way facts are manipulated but, in general, you are expected to construct some kind of argument. In this context, argument does not necessarily mean anything confrontational. It simply means that your essay should have a thread running through it.

Sometimes the wording of an essay title suggests a structure: *Discuss the effects of sex, age and social class in the development of asthma in Scotand.* This rather suggests a brief introduction, three, main, discursive, fact-presenting paragraphs and a brief closing paragraph.

If no obvious structure suggests itself, experiment with different ways of writing an essay plan.

Some people use mind maps. Put the core idea down on the middle of a bit of paper and let other ideas branch off. These secondary ideas might generate their own branches. Little clusters start to form. These might each form a section or paragraph of your argument. Do not worry if the same idea crops up in two places but ask yourself if that produces a possible link between sections.

You might prefer a more linear plan, like a flow chart, or you might try grouping related facts, listing pros and cons, and identifying major themes. These strategies may uncover such possible orders as: a logical progression as a proof unfolds, a chronological progression moving linearly backwards or forwards in time, a spatial structure, dealing with different geographic or topographic areas, a movement from the general to the particular, perhaps stating a hypothesis and testing it on specific examples, or moving from the particular to the general, constructing a hypothesis from the evidence you have set out.

If no plan emerges, do not despair. Sometimes the act of writing brings the necessary insights. Get started on freewriting. To do this, just write as fast as you can, without stopping to think, without lifting your pen, for at least three minutes. It doesn't matter if you write nonsense. At least you have something on paper to expand, re-order and improve.

If you still cannot see a way of making all the data hang together as a whole instead of a jumble of facts, seek help from your tutor.

FIRST DRAFT

The first sentence is always the hardest. A good way to tackle the opening paragraph is to put the question into your own words or say what you understand by it and prepare your reader for the way you are going to answer it. It will help your reader to understand your essay if you give an overview of where you are heading. You could state your objectives or list the main issues you intend to deal with (in the order that they appear in your essay) or say briefly what you intend to explain or discuss. In this opening paragraph, you want to get the reader on your side by arousing interest.

If you are having difficulty getting started, remember that you do not have to start at the beginning. Some of the ideas that you have jotted down whilst reading and note-taking can be written out to form a series of nuclei around which you can build up your text. Then you can fit them into your planned structure. If you prefer to write straight on to a word processor, a smaller window can be less intimidating than a huge blank screen waiting to be filled.

If the words still will not come, try talking. Explain what you are trying to write, to your flatmate, your cat or your bathroom wall. Write it down exactly as you said it.

Ideas are like buses – either none come or they all come at once. So, when you have plenty of ideas, just concentrate on getting them all down. Whether you use a word processor or pen and paper, just enjoy the experience. Worry about spelling, grammar, the exact words later. An essay which overflows with ideas and has to be refined is better than one that has to be padded out.

Stay flexible. What you write may give you new inspiration. You may find connections you had not noticed before and you may need to revise your essay plan a bit. It is very easy to move chunks of text around on your word processor; experimenting with structure is not a problem. However, when you move text around, make sure that the seams don't show. Read it over to check that the section you have moved links into its new surroundings.

The final paragraph should not introduce any new material or any new ideas. An old recipe for an essay structure is:

- Say what you are going to say.

- Say it.

- Say that you have said it.

This plan has been sneered at as over-simplified but there is a lot of sense in it. In particular, you will not go far wrong if your closing paragraph briefly restates the question and says how you have answered it. If you cannot show in your final paragraph that you have answered the question, perhaps you should ask yourself if you really have done so.

Make absolutely sure that everything you say is relevant. If necessary, point out why it is relevant. By now the essay title ought to be engraved on your heart. But just check again to make sure you have not lost sight of it. Is your essay a discussion, a comparison, or evidence in support of a hypothesis? Is that what was asked for?

Check for the following trademarks of woolly thinking:

- When you use a pronoun, can you identify the exact word or phrase it replaces? *This*, *these*, *that* and *those* are real danger words. After a long ramble, students often write, 'This means . . .' when it is not at all clear what 'this' was. An extreme example is afforded by a letter to the DSS: *I have not received any money from you. I have six children. Can you tell me why this is?*

- Be careful when starting a sentence with an *-ing* word or an *-ed* word. Make sure that the *-ing* or *-ed* word really does relate to the subject of the sentence or you could end up with nonsense like
    Walking down the main street, the parish church comes into view.
    Covered in a warm travelling rug, the coach bore him off into the night.

- Make absolutely certain that you have not missed out any steps in your argument.

By now you should really be confident that you understand your material and it is time to pass that understanding on to your reader as effectively as possible.

POLISHING

Effective communication is what makes good writers stand out. When you are writing essays, it is very easy to fall into the trap of thinking that this is between you and the page and you forget that a real person is going to have to read it and perhaps even enjoy it. Consider your reader.

Your reader is a well-informed academic who is going to take you and your essay seriously. The style is therefore formal. This does not mean that it has to be long-winded. It is very often the people who understand their subject best who can explain it most simply and directly. Those who have only half a grasp of what they are talking about are the ones who are most likely to dress up their shallow knowledge in dense language. They think they know what they want to say, but when it comes to putting it down on paper, the words won't come because they have not thought everything through. If you can say what you mean with absolute clarity, you will demonstrate your knowledge effectively. Look at every single sentence you write and ask yourself whether it is crystal clear. Trying to achieve this clarity will often expose a lack of understanding on your part and that is what makes essay writing such a good learning opportunity. You expose the gaps and work on them. Do not be tempted to fudge.

Murphy's Law of Writing: if your readers can misunderstand something they will. (And Murphy was an optimist.)

PREPARING FOR SUBMISSION

A departmental style sheet telling you how to set your work out is often given in a class booklet. If not, here are a few suggestions:

1. Make sure your typeface is big enough:
   - You could use 8 pt for footnotes at a pinch.
   - but 10 pt is just about the limit that older eyes can read comfortably for any length of time.

- 12 pt is easy on the eye (especially for ageing academics who have a lot of essays to read).
2. A page with plenty of white space is more attractive than a black, solid block of text. Make sure you use big margins so that the marker can write helpful comments. Separate your paragraphs with a blank line instead of indenting.
3. Imaginative use of fonts may help to make a point but, for the main body of your text, avoid weird and wonderful fonts.

FOOTNOTES OR ENDNOTES

Your departmental style sheet may give a ruling on this. If not, try to do whatever helps the reader. It is an irritation constantly having to flick to the end of a text. On the other hand, too many footnotes on a page can make for a very ugly appearance. For a few short notes which are important to the understanding of the text, the foot of the page is best. If they are copious and more for form than necessity, tuck them away at the end.

REFERENCES AND BIBLIOGRAPHIES

The purpose of references and bibliographies is to enable your readers to find for themselves the material to which you have referred. They may want to check your accuracy or, more positively, they may be stimulated by your writing to go and find out more. Whenever you are picking up another author's idea, even if you are not using the exact words, it is usual to use the author's surname, the date of publication and the page number in brackets (Wiseman, 1999, p. 999) after the citation or, if the author's name is part of your text, just bracket the date and the page number: Wiseman (1999, p. 999) is a fictitious example. If an author has more than one publication of the same date, these are designated 1999a and 1999b, etc.

Proper referencing is essential if you are not to be accused of plagiarism.

Plagiarism, whether intentional or unintentional, is a form of cheating which universities are very concerned about and they are increasingly vigilant to ensure that students do not copy work from other students, from published sources or from the internet. There are even computer programs designed to detect plagiarism. Of course you will present and discuss other people's ideas, opinions and theories in your essay, but you must say where you found them and you must be very careful not to claim them as your own original thoughts.

Bibliographies are a horrible chore, but the task can be made a lot easier if you note all the necessary information right from the very beginning of your research. It is soul-destroying chasing round libraries looking for things like page numbers and place of publication when the rest of the job is done.

The perfectionist will ensure that the latest editions of books are consulted wherever possible, but, if you cannot get hold of the most recent edition, list in your bibliography the one that you actually referred to.

If you are referring to a website, you must make sure that you give enough information to make sure that a reader could access the same site. Give the date in case the site has been updated since you used it.

The exact formats for bibliographies vary greatly and attention should be paid to where stops, commas and so on are used. If there is no set format, these are possible options:

Author, A. N. (1995) *Book Title in Italics*, Place: Publisher.
Author, A. N. (1996a) 'Article title without capitals', *Italicised Journal Name*, 10 (3): 1–55.
Author, A. N. (1996b) 'An essay in a book', in S. Cribble (ed.) *Book Title*, Place: Publisher.

PROOF-READING

Always proof-read on a hard copy. You will need to proof-read several times because you cannot do all the tasks at once.

Stage one

Take a break. It is very difficult to proof-read your own work and the more of a distance you can put between writing and rereading the better.

Stage two

Read for general sense and good communication. Read it out loud. Are there any bits that are unclear, get your tongue in a twist or sound rather pompous? At this stage, do not stop to correct things or you will lose the big picture. Just make a mark in the margin. Have you got the balance right, spending most time on the most important points? Once you have read right through, wrestle with the awkward sentences. Be careful that any improvements you make do not introduce new errors. When you are sure you have done everything for your reader that you would like an author to do for you, you may proceed to the next stage.

Stage three

Do the mechanical bits in turn. Use the spell checker but do your own check for things that it will miss like *it's/its*, *where/ were*. A very common kind of mistake is to mistype the little words, *on* instead of *of* for example. Is your punctuation helpful? Work out all the sums, double-check names and dates, physically look up everything that you have cross-referenced. When checking your grammar, common errors to look out for include verbs changing tense and pronouns drifting between *one* and *you*, sentences without verbs, run-on sentences where there should be a full stop in the middle, singular verbs with plural subjects and singular subjects with plural verbs.

Stage four

Give it to someone else to read, not necessarily a specialist in your subject. Ask them to make sure they can completely understand every sentence. In this way, they will test your own understanding. (Offer to do the same for them. You can learn a lot about your own writing from helping to make other people's writing clearer.)

Have a well-earned rest and look forward to an excellent mark. Then, when you get your essay back, resist the temptation to put it away in a file. Look at the comments carefully. If a few of you can get together and read each other's essays after marking you get a much better understanding of what makes a good essay in your subject.

NURSING ESSAYS ARE SPECIAL

You may be surprised to discover that, at least in the first year of a university course in nursing, students are not expected to be particularly innovative. There is a lot of groundwork to be learnt before you are ready to produce original work. Occasionally, students are worried because they feel they are not writing anything new but just reproducing what they have heard in lectures and read in books and articles, but essay writing in nursing is much more than just mindless copying out of facts. What the marker is looking for is the ability to handle all the information, to select the bits that answer the question and to put them together in a meaningful way. If you can do all that, you are demonstrating an understanding of the subject. Where you can use creativity and originality is in your selection of examples to illustrate the points you are making. If your examples are apt, the marker knows you have understood the concepts you are illustrating.

As you can see from the first part of this book, nursing embraces subjects of very different kinds. Some of them lend themselves to a very black and white, factual approach (e.g. physiology and anatomy) and others allow for more discussion (e.g. social sciences). If you are more familiar with the discussion type of essay, you may think it an easier option, but this is not necessarily true. If you are answering on physiology, you will not gain many marks for personal anecdotes; you must support your discussion of relevant points with accepted scientific evidence. The content of the lecture courses will give you insights into what is relevant and important.

If you think you have a tendency to waffle, chose an essay topic that focuses you on factual material. Again, the lectures are the best guide as to what to concentrate on.

COMPLETE DISASTER

What do you do if, in spite of all the good advice in this book, you fail to hand your essay in on time? You may have a good reason, such as illness. If so, you should provide a medical certificate. Your director of studies or personal tutor should be notified of serious personal problems which interfere with your work and they may be taken into account if you find you need an extension. Having three essays to hand in for the same day does not constitute grounds for an extension. It is merely a fact of university life and a very good reason for organising your time wisely. As soon as you feel you are behind schedule, have a word with your tutor.

If the worst comes to the worst, face up to it. Go to your tutor, lecturer or course organiser, own up and apologise. The longer you leave it, the harder it will be. Do *not* try to explain how your hard disk ate your essay at the last moment: you should have kept a floppy copy. *Nobody* believes that computers crash two hours before the submission time. By that late hour you should have a copy already printed out for a final proof-read. You could hand that copy in if the computer crashes. Better to hand in a late draft than a draft late. You may find that you will be marked down for late submission but, if you have ignored all this advice, that is exactly what you deserve!

WRITING A CARE STUDY

Nursing students will often be required to write care studies as part of their assessment programme. Unlike exam questions or essays in nursing, which are usually based on imaginary patients, a care study is usually based upon an actual person the nurse has looked after.

There are many regulations set out by various institutions regarding the conduct of care studies. The most important relate to guarding the individual's confidentiality and well-being. Every patient has the right to confidential treatment. It is a serious infringement of that right if an individual can be identified from a care-study report, perhaps because it may have been mislaid or left open in a library.

In most universities it is a requirement that students change the chosen patient's name. All information regarding address, date of birth, hospital number or anything else that may reveal the identity of a patient should be anonymised in all care studies. Student nurses should ensure to choose an appropriate patient for their care study. First that patient must give his or her consent to be the subject of a care study. The purpose of the study should be clearly explained to the patient and he or she should also be reassured that the only person to see the study will be the university tutor and that anonymity will be maintained at all time.

Permission to review the patient's nursing and medical notes should be obtained. Although the main objective in most nursing care studies is to enable the student nurse to fully understand the nursing care a patient receives, it also facilitates identification of other facets of health-care. A care study may provide a rationale for prescribed drugs and demonstrate the role of other health professionals in the health-care team.

As with the other types of written work addressed in this section there are certain factors that require clarification prior to writing a care study. These can be summarised as:

- Title: is there an exact title to the care study (e.g. 'Nursing care in stroke patients')?

- Word count: many university departments specify word ranges in written assessments.

- References: students should be aware of the in-house rules and regulations for referencing.

- Social history: nurses should appreciate the importance of social history in nursing care studies.

- Models of nursing: as discussed earlier in this book, nursing care is often based upon a specific nursing model. This should include a rationale for the model chosen and it should be based upon the nursing process.

- Demographic details: these should include age, family background and employment.

- Care setting: was the study conducted in the home or hospital?

- Additional information: information on medical investigations, relevant medical history, pathophysiology and current treatment will all contribute towards care study.

Student nurses may wish to include an appendix to their care study (i.e. a copy of their patient's nursing observation chart or their drug kardex, remembering to ensure the patient's anonymity).

Care studies in nursing enable students to view their patients as individuals, with their own background, problems and needs.

OTHER KINDS OF WRITING

Essays are the most demanding pieces of writing that you will be asked to do in first year. In later years, you may be asked to do a much longer dissertation and you may even want to write papers for conferences or articles for publication. Essay writing trains you for these activities. The processes are just the same. If you keep the needs of your reader in mind, you will be able to write for all occasions.

Do:

- Make yourself comfortable in a distraction-free zone.

- Use mind maps, flow charts and so on to help you make plans.

- Start writing as soon as you start researching.

- Try free writing or talking to get started or to unblock you if you get stuck.

- Ask for help if you need it.

FURTHER READING

P. Creme and M. Lea's *Writing at University: A Guide for Students* (1997), Open University Press, Buckingham, is a very approachable general introduction to university writing.

The Student's Guide to the Internet 1998/9 by I. Winship and A. McNab (1998), Library Association Publishing, London, is very helpful and easy to use but will date very quickly; keep an eye open for updated versions.

12 IMPROVING WRITTEN COMMUNICATION

As you progress through university, you will have to deal with more and more complex concepts and your teachers will demand ever more exacting standards of precision and accuracy. Such rigour in your thinking will be reflected in your writing style. Here are a few hints on how to achieve depth without sacrificing clarity in your academic writing.

PARAGRAPHS

Topic sentences

You should have one topic or core idea per paragraph. It is a good idea to summarise it in a topic sentence.

The best place for the topic sentence is at the beginning of the paragraph because it makes for easy reading if your reader knows what you are writing about. If your reader is scanning through your work, the first sentence of each paragraph will catch the eye. You can put it at the end, which is also a position which gives emphasis, but that makes it harder work for the reader. Of course, if you really want to drive a point home, you can put it at both beginning and end.

As you write, keep your topic sentence in mind. When you find yourself straying from it, you should be on to the next paragraph.

Conversation

When you are writing, you are holding a conversation without being able to hear the other person. At the end of each paragraph, in a conversation, your partner would come in with a comment like:

> *What happened next?*
> *Could you give me an example?*
> *You have given me a whole lot of examples. Are you going to imply something?*
> *Ah, but what if . . . ?*
> *Are there any other ways of looking at this?*
> *Say that again another way. I didn't understand a word of it!*

If your paragraphs are well planned, your reader should be coming to the same conclusion as you, just milliseconds before you state what has just become obvious. Or, at least, he or she will be formulating the question which your next paragraph is just about to answer. If you have experienced this in your reading, you will know how good it makes a reader feel.

Linking

In the best writing, one paragraph naturally and necessarily flows on to the next. Between paragraphs, take time to reflect:

• What did I establish in the last paragraph?

• How does my next paragraph relate to it?

In case the relationship is not immediately clear, it is helpful to have a few strategies ready to help you link paragraphs to each other.

For example, you could start with a paragraph which lists the topics to be discussed in the following paragraphs. You could end with a paragraph that summarises the preceding paragraphs. That may not be appropriate, if you are trying to follow an argument from beginning to end, in which case it might be helpful to have some signals ready to link paragraphs:

Enumerative:　*First . . . Second . . . Finally . . .*

Additive:　*Another example . . . Furthermore . . . Moreover . . .*

Contrastive:　*By contrast . . . On the one hand . . . On the other hand . . . Alternatively . . .*

When you are reading, make a note of any links which you think are effective and which you would feel comfortable using.

Beware, however, of overusing any of these links as they can easily become intrusive and irritating. Watch your writing very carefully for links that are becoming too much of a habit. *However* is one that many people pepper their work with.

The length of paragraphs should be varied. A long paragraph is hard reading and it is good to put in short, signpost ones, just to say where you have got to or where you are going, if you think you might be overloading your reader. The more important the point, the longer the paragraph, but an occasional, very short, punchy paragraph can be used very effectively to hammer home a vital point.

SENTENCES

The important thing about sentences is to keep the words in the right order. Do not alter the natural word order for rhetorical effect unless you really know what you are doing and you are really sure that your meaning will be made more rather than less clear.

The subject of the sentence goes at the beginning. It is no accident that the grammatical 'subject', the one that 'does' the verb, goes before the verb. The subject is what the sentence is about and the rest of the sentence is saying something about the subject. The second most conspicuous position in a sentence is at the end. Occasionally, it can be effective to build up to a climax at the end of a sentence.

A sentence is as long as it needs to be. If you are building complex relationships, your sentence might have to be very long but, if you keep the structure simple, a long sentence does not have to be difficult. Do not try to tuck too many additional bits of information into a sentence or your reader will loose the main thread. Too many short sentences sound rather ugly and fail to develop links and relationships but the very occasional short, sharp sentence can give a dramatic emphasis. Try to give your reader a bit of variety of sentence length.

Be impersonal . . .

. . . but know when to take responsibility for your own actions and opinions. Departments, and even individual lecturers, vary in their acceptance of the use of *I* in academic writing, but there is an increasing awareness outside universities that the use of the passive is a way of avoiding responsibility. 'The report could not be submitted before the meeting' actually means 'Oops, I missed the deadline'. When you want to make it clear that you are voicing a purely personal opinion, *I* is not only appropriate but essential: *It might be thought that . . . > I think . . .* (Not: *The author thinks . . .*)

Be active

Using the passive is a way of avoiding the use of *I*, but there is so much of the passive in academic prose that it becomes wearisome. Therefore, avoid it if you can.

It has been suggested by Smith . . . > Smith has suggested . . .

Be positive

Negatives can overstretch your readers' logical abilities:

There are no conditions under which the machine will not operate.

The elements of English grammar are not beyond 60 per cent of students.

Pressure must not be lowered until the temperature is not less than 40°C.

Be brief

Word limits take into account the number of words necessary to deal with the set topic. Using unnecessary words for padding out or running over the limit does not make for a good essay or for pleasant reading. By how much can you shorten these examples?

A feature of much of this research is the illustration of . . .

There is continued, ongoing research . . .

Basically, the true facts may be said to be as follows: an undue and excessive proliferation of redundant and unnecessary modifiers and other repetitious or fairly weak insertions add very little or nothing to the meaningful impact of the discourse.

Be careful!

Sometimes you can be too brief:

Elephants do not require additional protection from buffalo.

Make sure that what goes together stays together:

Rabbit wanted for child with lop ears.

Sometimes you can say more than you intended:

The doctor said that he had never before seen this rare subcutaneous parasite in the flesh.

VOCABULARY

Jargon

One man's technical term is another man's jargon. In choosing your words, keep your target reader constantly in mind. When you are writing for your tutors and lecturers, you should be able to show that you have understood the technical terms and can use them correctly and appropriately.

Big words

Do not use big words where a little one will do the same job. If by *termination* you mean *end*, then use *end*. There is nothing to be gained by substituting *utilise* for *use*. There is a place for big words where they are the best ones to convey an accurate meaning, but they are not to be used unnecessarily for the sole purpose of sounding authoritative. You will just end up not knowing what you are talking about. Be especially self-disciplined about avoiding words whose meaning you are not completely sure about. Either consult a dictionary or use a word you know.

Formality

You need to maintain a certain level of formality. In selecting short, commonly used words, you must avoid any slang terms and colloquialisms.

PREMODIFIERS

The build-up of long, heavily premodified, fluency-impairing noun phrases is a common failing in academic writing.

This could be rephrased:

Too many adjectives before a noun often impair the fluency of academic writing.

More verbs

Verbs make your text bounce along. Nouns and adjectives and prepositional phrases describing nouns are solid and slow your reader down. If you can use more verbs and fewer adjectives and nouns, you will sound much less boring:

After expulsion of the breath by the lungs . . .
After the lungs expel the breath . . .

You can increase the proportion of verbs to nouns by rewriting phrases like

make an adjustment to > adjust
come to the conclusion > conclude

Other examples which can be shortened to a single verb include:

arrive at a decision
make an examination of
conduct an investigation into

INFERENCE

In a real conversation, there is a lot of creativity coming from both sides. How many interpretations can you put on the following?

Where was I?
Are you on the phone?

These sentences work in conversation because you can rely on inference. You can give signals with your own facial expressions and other gestures. You alter your tone of voice. If an appropriate, unambiguous inference cannot be made, your hearer will ask what you mean. You can see if there is a blank or bewildered or angry or approving expression on a hearer's face. You can ask little 'tag' questions just to make sure the conversation is going as you intend. Right? When you write, you are deprived of all these safety checks.

You cannot assume that just because your reader is an expert in the subject, he or she will know what you mean anyway and reconstruct some sense from your half-expressed musings.

RHETORIC

Figures of speech are more likely to be found in writing where the purpose is to persuade or entertain than in the dispassionate prose of academic discourse. They should be used sparingly, but there are a few good tricks which are useful for getting your point across.

1. Simile

If you are going to use similes, chose ones which are really vivid. If you describe a parasite as looking *like a courgette seed*, you need to be sure your readers are readily familiar with courgette seeds.

2. Repetition

Usually, you go to quite a lot of effort to vary your sentence structure. A deliberate repetition of a pattern can therefore attract and hold the reader's attention.

> *I came. I saw. I conquered.*

Why do bears, wishes and Billy Goats Gruff always repetitively come in threes? The universality of the number three in folklore testifies to its power. Here is another triplet:

> *Some books are to be tasted, some to be swallowed whole and some few to be chewed and digested.* (Francis Bacon)

Here, the third time comes with a little extra. This is repetition and variation. Good writers have always exploited this device. Think of repetition with variation as the delivery of some weakening punches followed by the knock-out blow.

3. Rhetorical question

This can be very irritating if it is over-used. A useful strategy is to use a question as a topic sentence to open a paragraph, and then go on to answer it.

4. Climax

For maximum impact, make points in increasing order of importance so that the reader's interest grows to a peak. If you do it the other way round, the reader will be bored by mid-sentence. Similarly, always give your weakest examples or weakest arguments first and save the best for last.

PROFESSIONAL SPELLING

Spelling mistakes create a bad impression especially when you make mistakes with technical terms specific to your subject; you undermine your readers' faith in your professional ability. Use your spell checker to teach yourself spelling. If a word keeps coming up, take a moment to learn it. The academic writer always has a good dictionary to hand and uses it.

PUNCTUATION

Punctuation is not there for decoration but to help the reader. Too much punctuation can get in the way of fluent reading and if you put a piece of punctuation in the wrong place, it is obvious that you do not know what you are doing, whereas if you leave a piece of punctuation out it looks like a little typing error. The lazy student will therefore follow the maxim: when in doubt, leave it out, and even the skilful student will use punctuation economically.

Full stops

Between the capital letter and the full stop there should be one, and only one, complete statement.

Commas

Commas separate lists. Note that there is no comma before the *and* in British English.

The colours of the rainbow are red, orange, yellow, green, blue, indigo and violet.

Commas separate out non-essential bits (essential in upper case):

Suddenly, THE DOOR SLAMMED.
Because the door slammed, THE MAID SCREAMED.
Meanwhile, back at the ranch, TONTO WAS, *with great skill,* MAKING PANCAKES.

Note how commas can change meaning. Compare

The chainsaw jugglers, who had been drinking before the show, beheaded themselves.

with

The chainsaw jugglers who had been drinking before the show beheaded themselves.

In the first sentence, the bit in commas is an optional extra and all the jugglers in the sentence lost their heads. In the second sentence, the beheaded jugglers are limited to those who had been drinking. Think about the effect of adding commas to:

The students who are good at punctuation do well in their essays.

If a section in commas is, as here, in the middle of the sentence, make sure your commas come in pairs.

Brackets

They come in pairs too.

Dashes

Dashes can be used in much the same way as commas and brackets, for sectioning off an optional extra, but they should not be used to hang afterthoughts on to the end of sentences.

Brackets and dashes can be useful if commas start nesting. Compare

Bad writers, who frequently compose long-winded sentences, rendered, as this example shows, incomprehensible, more or less, to the average or even skilled reader, by the interpolation of little, badly positioned, extra bits, should be ostracised by the academic community.

with

Bad writers (who frequently compose long-winded sentences, rendered   as this example shows – incomprehensible to the average, or even skilled reader, by the interpolation of little, badly positioned, extra bits) should be ostracised by the academic community.

The second version is still dreadful, but not quite so nightmarish as the first.

Semicolons

If you feel that two sentences are so closely linked that you want to draw attention to the fact, you can use a semicolon instead of a full stop:

The students got very high marks; nothing in their answers was irrelevant to the question.

Semicolons are also useful for lists where the items consist of more than one word, especially if the individual items contain commas:

I shared a flat with three exotic dancers from a Paris nightclub; a large, brown rat, who snored; a highly intelligent, but eccentric, philosophy student, called Alfie, who had a pet snake called Lucy; an ex-politician; and several cockroaches.

Colons

You will notice how colons are used to introduce lists and examples in this book. They are also used to introduce quotations when no verb of saying is present.

Exclamation marks

Avoid them! They have very little place in academic discourse. And never, never, *never* use more than one at a time.

Hyphens

These can be useful for resolving ambiguities. Consider the difference between

extra-marital sex and extra, marital sex.

Hyphens should also be used to avoid weird spellings: *de-ice* rather than *deice* and *go-between* rather than *gobetween.*

If you are not sure whether a compound word is hyphenated or not, and you cannot find it in your dictionary, make a decision and stick to it.

Quotation marks

Use quotation marks for short quotes but do not use them for 'iffy' words. If you think a word is not quite consistent with your formality level, find an 'un-iffy' word instead.

Apostrophes

Apostrophes are the punctuation marks that people seem to find hardest. In fact, they are really easy. In very formal writing, you will not use apostrophes for shortened words. *Do not write don't. It's it is, isn't it?*
Apostrophes are used to show possession:

If the possessor is singular, use *'s* (*the queen's crown*)
If the possessor is plural and ends in -*s*, use *'* (*cats' tails*)
If the possessor is plural and does not end in -*s*, use *'s* (*men's heads*)
In other words, make the plural first and the possessive second.

Special care is needed with personal names ending in -*s* like *Robert Burns* and *Charles Dickens*. There is a convention which allows these names just to have an apostrophe: *Burns' poems*, although *Burns's* possessive form may also be made safely in the usual way by adding *'s* after the complete surname. It is a common mistake to put the apostrophe inside the name: *Dickens' books* are famous, but *Dicken's books* have been written by the less well-known Mr Dicken.
If the possessor is a pronoun, do not use an apostrophe. You would never dream of writing *hi's*, would you? The same goes for *its*. *His head. Its tail.*
This is not all that there is to say about punctuation, but it might be enough to prevent the commonest errors. When checking your punctuation, the question to ask yourself is always, 'Does it help the reader?'

FUTHER READING

In addition to a good dictionary and thesaurus, you might like to invest in one or two of the following, or find them in the library:

Hart's Rules for Compositors and Readers at the University Press Oxford (1983 edn) is a compact manual with all you will ever need to know about abbreviations, capitals, hyphens, italics, numerals, quotations, symbols, foreign phrases and so on. It also has widely used proof-reading symbols. Every professional academic writer should have one on his or her desk.

G. J. Fairburn and C. Winch get down to detail in *Reading, Writing and Reasoning* (1996) Buckingham: Open University Press. This is an excellent book.

J. Peck and M. Coyle provide help with the mechanics of writing in *The Student's Guide to Writing: Spelling, Punctuation and Grammar* (1999) Basingstoke: Macmillan.

Philip Gaskell combines a useful summary of the basics of good writing with some well-chosen examples of different styles in *Standard Written English* (1998) Edinburgh: Edinburgh University Press.

R. Quirk and S. Greenbaum's *A University Grammar of English* (1973) Harlow: Longman, is a useful book to refer to on occasion.

The Chicago Manual of Style (1993) Chicago: University of Chicago Press, is widely used as a standard reference book. It covers bookmaking and all you are ever likely to need on production and printing as well as giving a comprehensive and authoritative ruling on all matters of style.

WRITING SKILLS SELF-ASSESSMENT

When you have completed a piece of work, measure it up on the table below. Note down your strengths and weaknesses. Now and again when you write, look back on your comments on earlier work. Have you taken your own criticisms on board?

First impression:
  Layout
  Word processing
  Attention to detail

Content:
  Definitions
  Adequate research
  Argumentation
  Evaluation
  Balance of argument
  Fairness of presentation
  Answering the question
  Overall integrity of structure

Paragraphs:
  Length
  Signposting
  Conversation
  Linking

Sentences:
  Length
  Clarity
  Grammar

Vocabulary:
  Consistent formality
  Accuracy
  Clarity

Spelling:

Punctuation:
  Accuracy
  Helpfulness

Other comments:

---

13 EXAMINATIONS

PREPARING FOR EXAMS

Look at past papers

Read the instructions. How many questions are you going to be asked? How many topics have you covered? How many topics do you need to revise? There may well be some bits of the course that you find easier or more absorbing than others. These are the ones to concentrate on. Just make sure that, if you are question spotting, you cover a safe amount of material. It is a good idea to have at least one spare topic in the bank in case one of your chosen subjects does not come up or the question is asked in a way you don't like.

Pick your questions carefully

If you have a talent for biological and social sciences and have worked hard all through the course, you will do well whatever questions you pick, but, if you lack confidence, there are some questions types that can help you. It is possible to do really badly in an exam essay if you misread the question or wander off the point. You cannot stray from the point with biology questions, like questions 6 and 7 in the sample exam paper in Appendix I. With questions like these, you can see exactly where the marks are coming from. The same applies to sectioned, short-answer-type questions (like question 10). You might be asked for a definition of something you are not sure about, but you might manage to find something sensible to say about it and even if you do not, you can still get 80 per cent for getting all the rest right. You cannot get less than zero, so it is always worth making an attempt at an answer.

Plan your revision

You should be able to go over all your selected topics several times. Instead of planning to do one topic to death before going on to the next, aim to revise all your exam question topics once and then revise them all again, and again. That way, everything gets a fair turn and nothing gets skimped.

Revise

Instead of just reading over your notes, which can put you to sleep or make you think you're learning when you're not, try making notes of your notes and notes of the notes of your notes until you are down to a postcard's worth or less for each question. Then, check that you can expand it all again to exam-answer size. A glance at these notes before you go into the exam will give you all the confidence you need.

Do past papers

You might like to brainstorm a few past papers with friends to get ideas on how to structure answers, and at some point, when you are far enough on with your revision, but well before the examination date, set yourself a paper under exam conditions. The most frequently asked question is 'How much should I write?' and this is the best way to find out. How well can you fit your answers to the time allowed for each question? (See next paragraph.) You may be able to do exercise-type questions in less than the allotted time. Essay-type questions and definition-type questions, however, should take up all the time allowed. If you run out of things to say, you will have to go back to the books. Always learn more than you need, to allow for all the things that go straight out of your mind under the stress of the exam.

Do your sums

Three hours. Four questions. Three-quarters of an hour per question (maximum). Allow time for admin. (like writing your name on each answer book), reading each question carefully, reading question again even more carefully, planning your answer. Forty minutes' writing time, maximum.

9.30 a.m.	Start
10.05 a.m.	Think about finishing first question
10.15 a.m.	Finish first question
10.50 a.m.	Think about finishing second question
11.00 a.m.	Finish second question
11.35 a.m.	Think about finishing third question
11.45 a.m.	Finish third question
12.20 p.m.	Think about finishing fourth question
12.30 p.m.	Smile.

Calculations during exams to make the most of your timing are suggested in the hints on answers.

Look at more past papers

Now that you have the information needed to answer the questions, think how you would manipulate what you know to fit the different ways the questions are worded.

Make sure you know where and when the exam is

If you are not a morning person, get an alarm call or ask someone to see that you are up in time. You might be surprised by the number of people who sleep in on an exam morning.

ON THE DAY

(If you are unable to attend an exam, you must give your reason to the course organiser as soon as possible. If the reason is illness, you must produce a medical certificate.)

Get there in plenty of time so that you arrive feeling calm and confident, but do not get there too early; you do not want to hang about with a crowd of hysterical people working themselves into a nervous frenzy. Be sure you have everything you need: identification if required, watch, spare pens, handkerchief. If you want to, take a last look at your postcard-sized notes just to remind yourself that you really do know a lot. When you go into the examination hall, you will be asked to leave your notes, your coat and your bags at the back of the hall. Be sure to take your purse or your wallet with you.

The best cure for exam nerves is the knowledge that you have studied to the best of your ability. Remind yourself that you are as well prepared as you will ever be and look forward to showing off your knowledge. The examiners want you to pass and they are actively looking to reward you for displaying relevant knowledge. They are not going to try to catch you out. If nerves do begin to get the better of you, before or during the exam, breathe. Breathe very slowly and deeply, counting to seven (a lucky number) as you breathe in. Then see how slowly you can breathe out. Three breaths like this will have you perfectly calm.

Now read the instructions carefully. You will probably be asked to use a fresh examination book for each answer, Remember to put your name on each book, and your tutor's name if it is asked for.

If there is anything you need to ask the invigilator, just put your hand up. It does occasionally happen that misprints occur on exam papers, in spite of careful proof-reading. If something is missed out from the instructions, or they are not clear, the invigilator will be glad to hear about it and will inform the rest of the class. If you run out of paper, feel unwell, need to go to the toilet, or need to borrow a pen, put your hand up and the invigilator will come to you.

Read through the questions and choose the ones you are going to do. Decide on the order in which you are going to do them. Make a note of the time at which you will need to start drawing each question to a conclusion. Make a note of the time at which you stop doing each question, finished or not. Do not be tempted to overrun. Use any time left over to check through your answers, but do not start dithering and changing things that were right in the first place. If in doubt, go with your first instincts.

AFTER THE EXAM

When the exam is over, avoid people who ask, 'What did you write for question two?' It is over, finished, and there is nothing you can do to change it. Do not think about it again until you get the results. When you come out of an exam, you may still have a lot of left-over adrenalin. If you have two exams in one day, you need to come down to earth. Take a brisk walk, have something to eat and focus on the next exam.

When you get your exam back, even if you have done brilliantly, look at the examiner's remarks. Do you see where you went wrong?

Marks are most commonly lost because of:

- Not reading the instructions and doing one question too few or one too many.

- Not reading the question.

- Bad time management.

- Irrelevance.

- Trying to substitute made-up waffle for fact.

- Not giving enough examples.

Almost as importantly, do you see where and how you did well? Now you know what the examiners are looking for, make sure you give them more of it next time. Any problems, ask your tutor.

APPENDIX

SAMPLE DEGREE EXAM PAPER

This specimen paper is modelled on the kind of questions set at Edinburgh University. The actual content of the course is altered from time to time and other universities do not teach exactly the same things but it will give you some idea of the breadth of topics covered. There is something to appeal to every taste. If you are reading this before you start your course, remember that this is aimed at students who know a whole year's worth of nursing more than you do. It is not surprising that it looks quite hard in places. You will not find all the answers in this book. On the positive side, you will see that you really do have a wide choice of topics and you might even be able to tackle one or two of them already. Students sitting this exam will already know what topics they are best at and what type of questions suit them best.

This is a three-hour exam. Students must do FOUR questions from the following:

1. Explain why listening is more important than hearing.
2. Discuss how primary nursing humanises care in hospital.
3. Discuss the concept of role in relation to the health-care system.
4. Mental-health problems are caused by diseases of the brain. Discuss.
5. Describe the communication skills a nurse could use to help a patient talk about his or her anxieties.
6. Outline the structure of the respiratory tract and describe how ventilation is achieved.

7. Describe the principal events of a cardiac cycle.
8. Compare and contrast the routes of drug administration.
9. How do health promotion and health education differ?
10. Write short paragraphs to explain each of the following:
    a) nitrogen balance
    b) basal metabolic rate
    c) body mass index
    d) hypothalmic regulation of food intake.

REFERENCES

Alexander, M. F., Fawcett, J. N., and Runciman, P. J. (2000) *Nursing Practice: Hospital and Home*, Edinburgh: Churchill Livingstone.

Council for the Education and Training of Health Visitors (1977) *An Investigation into the Principles of Health Visiting*, London: CETHV.

Henderson, V. (1969) *The Basic Principles of Nursing Care*, Geneva: International Council of Nurses.

Roper, N., Logan, W., and Logan, A. (1985) *The Elements of Nursing*, 2nd edn, Edinburgh: Churchill Livingstone.

Royal College of Nursing (1995) *Whose Prescription?*, London: RCN.

Twinn, S., and Cowley, S. (1992) *The Principles of Health Visiting: A Re-examination*, London: Health Visitors' Association.

World Health Organisation (1985) *Targets for Health for All by the Year 2000*, Copenhagen: WHO.

INDEX